Evidence-based Healthcare: A
Therapists

Evidence-based Healthcare: A Practical Guide for Therapists

Edited by

Tracy J. Bury MSc MCSP
Head of Research and Development,
The Chartered Society of Physiotherapy,
14 Bedford Row, London, UK

Judy M. Mead MCSP
Head of Clinical Effectiveness,
The Chartered Society of Physiotherapy,
14 Bedford Row, London, UK

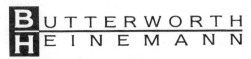

OXFORD   AUCKLAND   BOSTON   JOHANNESBURG   MELBOURNE   NEW DELHI

Butterworth-Heinemann
Linacre House, Jordan Hill, Oxford OX2 8DP
225 Wildwood Avenue, Woburn, MA 01801-2041
A division of Reed Educational and Professional Publishing Ltd

A member of the Reed Elsevier plc group

First published 1998
Reprinted 1999 (twice), 2000, 2001

British Library Cataloguing in Publication Data

A catalogue record for this book is available from the British Library

Library of Congress Cataloguing in Publication Data

A catalogue record for this book is available from the Library of Congress

ISBN 0 7506 3783 8

For information on all Butterworth-Heinemann publications
visit our website at www.bh.com

Typeset by E & M Graphics, Midsomer Norton, Bath
Printed and bound in Great Britain by The Bath Press, Bath

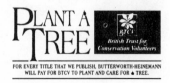

FOR EVERY TITLE THAT WE PUBLISH, BUTTERWORTH-HEINEMANN
WILL PAY FOR BTCV TO PLANT AND CARE FOR A TREE.

Contents

Foreword   vii
Preface   ix
List of Contributors   xi
Acknowledgements   xiii

Section I   BACKGROUND AND SCENE SETTING   1

Chapter 1   Evidence-based healthcare explained   3
             Tracy Bury

Chapter 2   Clinical effectiveness: another
             perspective to evidence-based healthcare   26
             Judy Mead

Section II   FACILITATING CHANGE   43

Chapter 3   Change management   45
             Jane Keep

Chapter 4   Getting research into practice: changing behaviour   66
             Tracy Bury

Chapter 5   Involving service users   85
             Gill Needham and Sandy Oliver

Section III   DEVELOPING AND APPLYING SKILLS   105

Chapter 6   Finding the evidence   107
             Andrew Booth and Bruce Madge

Chapter 7   Reading and critical appraisal of the literature   136
             Tracy Bury and Christina Jerosch-Herold

Chapter 8   Developing, disseminating and implementing
             clinical guidelines   162
             Judy Mead

Chapter 9   Implementing evidence through clinical audit   182
             Yvette Buttery

Section IV   THE WAY FORWARDS   209

Chapter 10   Making evidence-based healthcare happen   211
Judy Mead and Tracy Bury

Appendices

Appendix 1 Checklists for critical appraisal   227

Appendix 2 Useful information sources   235

Appendix 3 Acronyms   243

Index   245

Foreword

Evidence-based healthcare and evidence-based practice are familiar terms to most therapists and are considered worthwhile goals. Nevertheless, there is often uncertainty about their precise definition, who should be involved, what they should be doing and how to go about it. Therapists, like other healthcare professionals, have become suspicious of some topics that have been introduced into the National Health Service (NHS), especially those that have turned out to be management fads, requiring a high expenditure of time for little clinical gain. Evidence-based healthcare is not one of these danger zones. The amount of effort that we put in to improving our individual and collective efforts in this area will lead to improvements in patient care and in professional development.

Tremendous variations in clinical practice exist which are the result of individual therapists' skills, knowledge, experience and abilities, along with the resources, trends and philosophies of different service providers. These differences can lead to a lottery for the consumers. Patients will benefit most from seeing a skilled therapist who has integrated the latest evidence into his or her practice and has the backing of appropriate resources. However, this is not always the case and certainly is not an issue for therapy services alone.

The emphasis within the evidence-based movement is to ensure that consumers have a greater assurance that they are receiving care based on the best available evidence, wherever they go for their treatment. Effort expended on this topic would be worthwhile if only to achieve the best clinical care for patients. However, there are additional advantages. Each practitioner will feel a greater professional pride and confidence as he or she undertakes his or her tasks. Furthermore, professional bodies will have greater certainty with regard to the practice of their members and confidence in representing their profession, if they are assured that their contributions are clinically and cost-effective and of benefit to patients.

Working towards this more ideal state of care will not be without its difficulties. Virtually every aspect of a therapist's professional life will have to be touched. Continually updating and changing practice to reflect new, reliable research evidence, followed by monitoring and evaluation, are some of the basic requirements of using research. There will have to be cultural change and supporting infrastructure in order to achieve this across all sectors.

It may come as a surprise to some to learn that the move towards evidence-based healthcare involves not only practitioners and researchers, but all those concerned in the healthcare process, from policy-makers to users. All have roles and responsibilities that must be known, understood and implemented to achieve the desired goal and bring about this change.

This book addresses all of these issues in a straightforward and comprehensive manner, providing a clear explanation of what is involved for all parties concerned. It is a user-friendly step-by-step guide through the process. It offers a balanced discussion, acknowledging debates in other professions, and recognizes the individual and population perspectives that need to be considered. This reflects the emphasis on public health and the need to redress inequalities in healthcare. In doing this, it offers reassurance whilst recognizing the complexities. It will assist therapists by ensuring that they have the basic information, skills and tools required for evidence-based healthcare. In doing so, therapists will have the confidence that they not only must, but can be involved in helping to make all healthcare evidence-based.

Success in this respect is important. Evidence-based healthcare is not just a transient buzzword. It is an over-arching operational system that offers widespread benefits. Practitioners, managers and others will gain the additional confidence that accompanies an increased knowledge of the evidence base in their field and will use the evidence to provide optimal treatment. They will also acquire the tools with which to enter into partnerships with users and other professionals, to make shared decisions about appropriate interventions. This book provides information that will be useful to those involved in the move towards evidence-based healthcare, irrespective of their level of prior knowledge, experience or workplace setting. Read on, and turn the rhetoric of evidence-based healthcare into reality.

Professor Pam Enderby, PhD, FRCSLT
Dr Irene Ilott, PhD, SROT
Professor Di Newham, PhD, MCSP

Preface

Evidence-based healthcare and clinical effectiveness, relatively new terms within healthcare, have become everyday words. Implicit is the intention to do more good than harm for patients and ensure quality services, based on the best available evidence. This has been largely embraced within healthcare, although some suspicion and scepticism remains.

During the writing of this book, UK government policy has increased its commitment to evidence-based healthcare and there is nothing to suggest that this will lessen over the coming years. Also, there has continued to be an increasing number of papers written on the subject of evidence-based healthcare. By the time this guide reaches the bookshelves there will have been more published and more debate. However, it has been written to provide you with broad principles and tools that you can apply now. Also, because of the emphasis on change management, you should be well equipped to deal with any information which might impact on evidence-based decision-making in the future.

Why a book for therapists? Each profession has its own dynamics which can influence how similar issues are translated in practice. Much of the debate has centred on medicine. However, we felt it was important to transfer this into the working lives of therapists. In doing so, it should be as applicable to a student beginning his or her professional life as to an established therapist. Many of the references and case studies used in the book have come from physiotherapy. This reflects the fact that more has been written in this area than in the other therapies, not necessarily that the discussions have been any less prolific or diverse. That said, the examples provided have been used to illustrate key issues and practical advice which should be applicable to all therapists and other health professionals.

The term **healthcare** has been used throughout to encompass social care, education, industry and any number of areas within which therapists work. This extends to the private, independent and voluntary sectors. Much of the work to date has focused on acute care settings, although this is changing and extending to other areas. The term **practitioner** has been used rather than **clinician** and **intervention** rather than **treatment**, as we feel that these are more inclusive. Contributors have been used to bring their knowledge and experience from a range of fields, recognizing the contribution of different perspectives in evidence-based healthcare.

The focus throughout has been on the UK healthcare system, which we realize misses the international perspective. However, there are different healthcare systems and incentives, which vary from country to country, such as medical insurance being a driving force in the USA. Much of the literature concerning evidence-based medicine originated in Canada and has been translated to a UK environment. Likewise, the principles and guidance offered in this book should still equip readers to make evidence-based decisions working in different countries.

The book is structured into four main sections. From the theoretical introduction in section I, you are prepared for the management of change in section II. This includes the essential need to collaborate and build partnerships with service users, an area which is only now beginning to evolve. Section III focuses on developing your skills, such as literature searching and critical appraisal, and guidance on applying the principles in practice through clinical guidelines and clinical audit. This should leave you well equipped to take forwards evidence-based healthcare, integrating theory with practice. The final section pulls together the main themes from the book and poses questions to assist you in this process.

There are no hard and fast rules for making this happen. You need to be prepared for a wide range of situations and decisions. It is not a book of answers, but it should equip you to take a flexible evidence-based approach to each individual situation.

Tracy J. Bury
Judy M. Mead

Contributors

Andrew Booth, BA, MSc, Dip. Lib. A.L.A.
Director of Information Resources, School of Health and Related Research (ScHARR), 30 Regent Street, Sheffield, UK

With 14 years experience in a variety of health information contexts, his current role has involved setting up a regional information resource for evidence-based practice. The author of the *ScHARR Guide to Evidence Based Practice* and the Netting the Evidence Web site, he has written extensively on finding the evidence.

Tracy Bury, MSc, MCSP
Head of Research and Development, The Chartered Society of Physiotherapy, London, UK

Has been with the Society since 1994, developing initiatives across all areas of research and development. This has included involvement with the Joint Therapies Research Group and work to establish priorities for physiotherapy research, following consultation with the profession, consumers and others. Member of the Advisory Board for the Cochrane Rehabilitation and Related Therapies Field. Previously worked as a chartered physiotherapist in back pain management and rheumatology.

Yvette Buttery, BA(Hons), MPH, RGN
Lead facilitator, Clinical Audit and Effectiveness, Luton and Dunstable Hospital NHS Trusts, Luton, UK

Has worked in the field of clinical audit since 1992, and more recently this has included clinical effectiveness. Involvement has been at national, regional and trust levels. This included, from 1993–5, an evaluation of clinical audit in the National Health Service in England.

Christina Jerosch-Herold, DipCOT, SROT, OTR, MSc
Senior Lecturer and Joint Undergraduate Course Director, School of Occupational Therapy and Physiotherapy, University of East Anglia, Norwich, UK

An occupational therapist teaching research methods and critical appraisal skills to undergraduate and postgraduate healthcare professionals. Involved in the interdisciplinary modular MSc in Health Sciences and evidence-based practice workshops for therapists.

Jane Keep, MSc, MIPD, MIMgt
Fellow, Health Services Management Centre, University of Birmingham, and Human Resources Policy, NHS Confederation, London, UK

Eighteen years working in management within the National Health Service. More recently, in coupling the NHS employers' organization with academia, she has been working on national human resource policy issues, managing, consulting, researching and writing on organizational development and change management.

Bruce Madge, A.L.A
Head of the Health Care Information Service, The British Library, London, UK

Has a background of working in healthcare libraries and informatics at a local and district level, before moving on to national positions with the British Medical Association and the British Library. Currently in charge of the UK input into MEDLINE and the AMED databases.

Judy Mead, MCSP
Head of Clinical Effectiveness, The Chartered Society of Physiotherapy, London, UK

A chartered physiotherapist, who has worked at the Chartered Society of Physiotherapy for a number of years, leading its work on quality, standard-setting and, more recently, clinical effectiveness and clinical guidelines. Previously regional audit coordinator in Oxford, where she also worked with the Critical Appraisal Skills Programme.

Gill Needham, BA Hons, DipLib, MScEcon
Subject Team Leader, Open University Library, Milton Keynes, UK

Her main interests have been in evidence-based healthcare and in sharing evidence with users. She was involved for a number of years with the Critical Appraisal Skills Programme and with consumer health information. Previously she was Research and Development Specialist with Buckinghamshire Health Authority. She is currently in a post at the Open University and acts as a consultant to the Centre for Health Information Quality.

Sandy Oliver, PhD
Research Officer, Social Science Research Unit, London University Institute of Education, and Honorary Visiting Fellow at the UK Cochrane Centre, Oxford, UK

Has brought a consumer perspective to the National Health Service research programmes through her membership of the National Childbirth Trust. She has worked with the Critical Appraisal Skills Programme and the NHS National Coordinating Centre for Health Technology Assessment. She has been exploring consumer contributions to research, and developing training and support for consumers who are planning or using research.

Acknowledgements

Many people have helped to inform and stimulate the ideas presented in this book. In particular, we would like to express our thanks to the Critical Appraisal Skills Programme (CASP) team in Oxford for the opportunity to be involved in and benefit from various developmental initiatives over a number of years.

In addition, our work at the Chartered Society of Physiotherapy, through workshops, strategy and policy development initiatives, and contact with members, has helped us to develop our thinking about the needs of therapists in preparing this book. In turn, this has led to further enhancements related to research and clinical effectiveness for the profession. This two-way process has provided a constant reminder of the complexities of practice and the need to keep ideas firmly grounded in reality.

The contributors' input was vital in ensuring that readers would be provided with an overall picture. They also commented on the whole book which helped to ensure continuity throughout. Individuals commented on various chapters and these are acknowledged within the book. In addition, Katrina Bannigan, Carol David and Jennifer Klaber-Moffett kindly looked at the whole book and provided valuable comments. Throughout the production of the book this advice has helped to enrich the content and make it as user-friendly as possible.

Finally, we would like to thank the many family members, friends and work colleagues who have provided support and encouragement through the peaks and troughs of this experience!

Background and Scene Setting

Evidence-based healthcare and clinical effectiveness are terms which have now become part of everyday practice for health professionals. It is important that if the opportunities offered by these developments are to be realized, a common understanding of the terms is reached. Ultimately they are about providing healthcare that does more good than harm, in terms of health gain and patient experience. Questioning how we know this to be the case means that decisions about healthcare become more explicit and accountable.

The healthcare environment is constantly changing and the views and needs of different stakeholders may result in competing demands. These need to be resolved and therefore it is important to understand each individual's role and responsibility in achieving this. This includes practitioners, managers, purchasers, policy-makers and consumers. Working together with common goals will ensure that the benefits of evidence-based healthcare and clinical effectiveness result in improvements for patient care and cost-effective services.

1

Evidence-based healthcare explained

Tracy Bury

What is evidence-based healthcare?

Evidence-based healthcare is one, if not **the** buzzword of 1990s healthcare, one which is open to interpretation and confusion. This chapter provides an overview of evidence-based healthcare in its widest sense. Does it create opportunities for improved patient care, or does it seek to threaten clinical autonomy with cookbook recommendations? To date, much of this debate has centred on evidence-based medicine. However, this is just one element of evidence-based healthcare. The broader term opens up the debate for all those involved in healthcare, whether practitioners, managers, providers, commissioners/purchasers, policy-makers or service users. Within the book, healthcare has been used to encompass all settings in which health professionals work, including social care, public health, health promotion and education, as well as the National Health Service (NHS), private, independent and voluntary sectors. In doing this, it recognised that therapists work in many settings and organizational structures that require inter-agency and inter-sector collaboration.

Background

The Department of Health launched its Research and Development (R&D) Strategy for the NHS in 1991 (Department of Health, 1991). In the opening paragraph, Sir Michael Peckham, the Director of R&D, clearly set out the primary objective of the strategy. He said that it was '... to see that R&D becomes an integral part of health care so that practitioners, managers and other staff find it natural to rely on the results of research in their day to day decision making and longer term strategic planning'. He added that, 'Strongly held views based on belief rather than sound information still exert too much influence in health care. In some instances the relevant knowledge is available but is not being used, in other situations additional knowledge needs to be generated from reliable sources'.

In setting out this objective, the role of research as integral to healthcare is clearly defined. The importance of research in informing the provision of healthcare is highlighted, as is the need to try to ensure that where sound evidence exists it is transferred to practice. In part this acknowledges the wide variations that exist in practice. Patients who present with very similar signs and symptoms can be treated in a variety of ways depending on who they see, or where they are seen (Gray et al, 1997).

Scope and definition

The scope of evidence-based healthcare is illustrated in Figure 1.1. It can be separated into key strands: evidence-based commissioning/ purchasing, evidence-based policy; evidence-based management; evidence-based patient choice, and evidence-based practice.

Evidence-based healthcare has been described as care that 'takes place when decisions that affect the care of patients are taken with due weight accorded to all valid, relevant information' (Hicks, 1997). In setting out this definition, supporting statements were provided to assist with interpretation.

- The **decisions** are seen to be those of managers, health policy-makers and practitioners. This should also include patients.

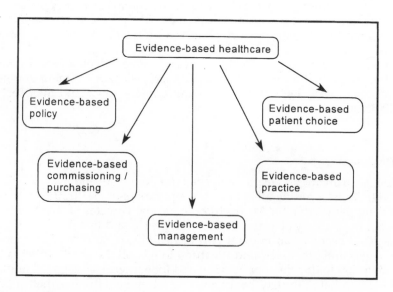

Figure 1.1 Evidence-based healthcare.

- **Due weight** infers that many factors contribute to decisions. Clinical and policy decision-makers, while using evidence from high-quality research, will also use information about patient preferences and resources. It does not assume that one sort of evidence should necessarily be the determining factor in a decision.
- The use of the word **all** is an aim, as it assumes an active and comprehensive search for relevant information.
- The term **information** is designed to be inclusive rather than exclusive. It requires that the **validity** (accuracy) and **relevance** (applicability) of each information source is assessed in the context of the decision.

On reading this, some would argue that evidence-based healthcare is not a new approach, so what is all the fuss about? Perhaps the question that should challenge everyone is: 'how do you know that what you do works?' While the approach may not be new, the emphasis on research-based evidence has increased. This is partly in response to the growth in research information, the recognition that more concerted efforts are required to implement high-quality research in practice, the organization of this information into more readily accessible formats, and advances in information technology (Gray, 1997).

From this discussion it can already be seen that evidence-based healthcare is about decision-making, a recurrent theme throughout this book. Ultimately it is about how the evidence, derived from a wide range of sources, can be incorporated into decisions that affect the care of populations and individuals.

Evidence-based practice is primarily about the interaction between a practitioner and an individual. Evidence-based patient choice can be at both an individual and a population level, especially if service users are used in healthcare planning. Evidence-based commissioning/purchasing and evidence-based policy are primarily concerned with populations and overall services. Evidence-based management should bridge the gap between individual and population perspectives. All aspects are interactive. The need to take account of both individual and population perspectives will be explored later in the chapter.

Evidence-based practice is the area with which therapists will be most familiar. However, in order to reflect the complexities of healthcare and the decision-making process, you will need to be acquainted with all facets. Depending on your position within an organization's structure, you will be more actively involved in some areas than others. Building partnerships with users to facilitate evidence-based patient choice is everyone's responsibility. Being proactive in preparing business or service specifications will fall to both providers and purchasers if evidence-based commissioning is to be successful. Managers will then have to put this into operation within the context of a whole service. The issue of evidence-based patient choice is covered in detail in Chapter 5. Evidence-based commissioning/purchasing, evidence-based policy and evidence-based management are dealt with in this chapter and are followed up in Chapter 2.

Defining evidence-based practice

The term **practice** encompasses areas relevant to specific professions or client groups (see Figure 1.2), each with its own dynamics and knowledge base.

To start to understand what evidence-based practice is, it is useful to refer to the debates concerning evidence-based medicine. Evidence-based medicine is defined as, 'the conscientious, explicit, and judicious use of current best evidence in making decisions about the care of individual patients.' (Sackett et al, 1996). Debates have centred on interpretation, or misinterpretation, of this definition. The definition alone stimulates such debates and it is important to explore its full meaning. This has been done to address particular elements of the definition (Haynes et al, 1996; Sackett et al, 1996) and the following sections explore this in detail. However, the issues raised are relevant to all aspects of evidence-based healthcare.

Sources of evidence

The term **judicious use** is seen to require the balancing of risks and benefits of alternative sources of evidence. These sources of evidence may include:

- Research evidence: derived from high-quality, systematic research
- Clinical expertise: from experience with patients, established practice, experts in the field, development of skills through continuing professional development
- Beliefs and values of the therapist and patient: based on previous

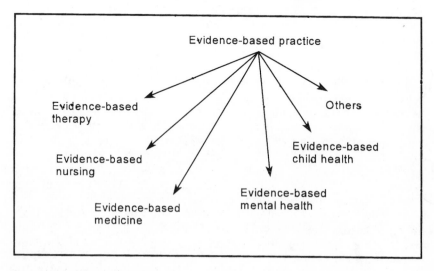

Figure 1.2 Evidence-based practice.

experience (e.g. of health services, of life), interactions and expectations, thereby introducing a social context
• Clinical assessment of the patient: information gathered
• Patients' preferences.

Evidence therefore encompasses a wide range of information sources, of which research evidence is just one. Many areas do not have a firm scientific research base. While research may not have shown interventions to be effective, this does not equate to evidence of ineffectiveness. The research may simply not have been done yet, it may have been of poor quality, or it may have produced inconclusive results. Therefore, limiting the type of evidence to that derived from research does not provide a decision-making model that is feasible or reflective of the complexity of practice.

What is 'best' evidence?

The use of the term **best evidence** primarily refers to scientific evidence derived from research. Specific questions need certain research methods to answer them. Therefore, in considering the scientific evidence, it is important to have defined the nature of your enquiry in order to track down the relevant research. There is not one single methodology that specifically addresses issues of effectiveness.

The process of research is aimed to:

• Generate new knowledge
• Provide results that are generalizable, i.e. which can be applied to similar patients and situations not included in the original study, for whom it is considered applicable
• Challenge the current situation or practice
• Inform policy and service delivery.

While one piece of research alone is unlikely to address all of these aims, they all form part of the healthcare 'jigsaw'.

Research has been described as falling into two categories (Gray, 1997):

1. That which increases the understanding of health, ill-health and the process of healthcare.
2. That which enables an assessment of the interventions used in order to try to promote health, to prevent ill-health or improve the process of healthcare.

The former concentrates on developing a knowledge base from which ideas can be generated for evaluation using the second category of research. It also provides contextual information against which the evidence arising from the latter should be interpreted. It is the second approach which is primarily concerned with the evaluation of ideas in practice.

Hierarchies of scientific evidence exist, based on the validity (accuracy) of different methodologies and the extent to which they can reduce the likelihood of errors in the conclusions reached and recommendations

Table 1.1 Hierarchy of strength of evidence

I	Strong evidence from at least one systematic review of multiple well-designed randomized controlled trials
II	Strong evidence from at least one properly designed randomized controlled trial of appropriate size
III	Evidence from well-designed trials without randomization, single group pre-post, cohort, time series or matched case-controlled studies
IV	Evidence from well-designed non-experimental studies from more than one centre or research group
V	Opinions of respected authorities, based on clinical evidence, descriptive studies or reports of expert committees

made. An example is presented in Table 1.1 (Moore et al, 1995). Do not worry if you are unfamiliar with some of the types of research mentioned, as they will be discussed further in Chapter 7.

When reviewing the evidence, the idea is to rank studies depending on the degree to which the observed results are likely to be attributable to the intervention being studied. It should be remembered that the hierarchy is based on high-quality studies being carried out in each category. A well-done cohort study will be more reliable than a poorly performed randomized controlled trial (RCT).

Why should systematic reviews be at the top of the list? First of all it is important to draw a distinction between systematic reviews and other types of reviews. While many **reviews** summarize the results from a number of studies and draw conclusions, they have often been produced without a thorough search for all the available studies. Also, individual studies may not have been quality assessed. A **systematic review**, however, uses explicit methods to 'identify, select and critically appraise relevant research', and to collect and analyse the data from individual studies (Mulrow and Oxman, 1997). This search for information is based on a clearly defined question.

Generally, systematic reviews can be used to answer most questions, whether they concern diagnosis, treatment, screening or managerial interventions, or focus on quality, acceptability or cost-effectiveness outcomes (Gray, 1997). They are one way of tackling the sheer volume of information that exists (Mulrow, 1994). It has been estimated that over two million articles about healthcare are published each year, scattered in over 20 000 biomedical journals (Ad Hoc Working Group for Critical Appraisal of the Medical Literature, 1987). If you were to stack these articles, they would reach a height of 500 metres (Mulrow, 1994). This just includes the information that finds its way into published sources. Systematic reviews also aim to track down information that does not result in a publication. They provide a way of focusing on high-quality material, drawing conclusions from previous work which may have proved inconclusive or conflicting (Mulrow, 1994; NHS Centre for Reviews and Dissemination, 1996). In doing so, they provide a clearer

bottomline about the degree of effectiveness of an intervention, which should help you in making decisions.

Randomized controlled trials are considered by many to be the next best approach to determining the effectiveness of many interventions. However, there is some concern that over-emphasis on the importance of RCTs belies the fact that other methods may be more suitable, depending on the question (Black, 1996). For example, it would not be ethical to undertake an RCT to examine the effectiveness of intensive care units. Also, imposing this medical gold standard of the RCT may be inappropriate in many areas of rehabilitation and therapy research (Andrews, 1991; Gladman, 1991).

The outcomes being investigated also need to be considered when deciding on the appropriateness of a research design (Gray, 1997). Again, systematic reviews will usually provide the strongest evidence. Where the outcome of interest is the acceptability of an intervention or service, qualitative, survey or RCT methodologies are appropriate. If the outcome is appropriateness then RCTs are not suitable, whereas qualitative or survey methods are (Gray, 1997). These examples illustrate that the question determines the method used.

Limiting the application of one hierarchy to determine the strength of the evidence does not accommodate the need for specific methods, depending on the research question. A hierarchy is only appropriate if it is tailored to the question being posed. If the question is about appropriateness then the hierarchy might look something like Table 1.2.

Invariably, in order to answer your question, it will be necessary to consider the scientific evidence derived from more than one type of research. Increasingly, research combines several methodological approaches in order to answer questions more comprehensively, taking into account the need for a range of outcome measures.

While the value of opinions is recognized within the hierarchy, it also acknowledges that where possible these should be based on evidence collected systematically from practice. Opinions will be biased by the experience and values of those involved and should therefore be treated cautiously, although in many areas of healthcare they are currently the best available evidence.

Individual patients and clinical expertise

Sackett and colleagues (1996) claim that more thoughtful identification and compassionate use of **individual patients' predicaments, rights and**

Table 1.2 Strength of evidence to answer questions of appropriateness

I	Strong evidence from at least one systematic review
II	Qualitative or survey study designs from more than one centre or research group
III	Opinions of respected authorities, including service users, based on experience, or reports of expert committees

preferences are reflected in greater decision-making expertise. In doing so they emphasize that external clinical evidence can inform, but never replace, individual **clinical expertise**. This expertise enables patients' rights and preferences to be incorporated into the decisions. Having a sound understanding and knowledge of a condition and underlying pathology allows you to interpret the evidence and determine its relevance to the individual patient (Evidence-Based Medicine Working Group, 1992). This process is vital, as the inclusion criteria restricting patients included in a research study often do not resemble your patient or take account of coexisting conditions. Only when you have decided that the external evidence applies to your individual patient can it be integrated into the clinical decision.

For each individual patient, the illness is unique in terms of his or her experience of it and the way it presents (Sullivan and MacNaughton, 1996). Patients have often reached conclusions about their problem before they seek advice and these need to be elicited. By listening to the patient and with appropriate questioning you can explore that patient's beliefs, their foundation and preferences. Understanding the patient's perspective is important for entering into a decision-making partnership.

Sackett and colleagues (1996) talked of the role of doctors in 'identifying and applying the most efficacious interventions to maximise the quality and quantity of life for individual patients'. Maynard (1997) challenged the use of the word 'apply' as it is seen to reinforce the authoritarian doctor role of doing something to patients, rather than involving patients as active participants in their care. This can be seen to be at odds with the notion of evidence-based patient choice. You will need to decide if the evidence applies to your patients by considering if

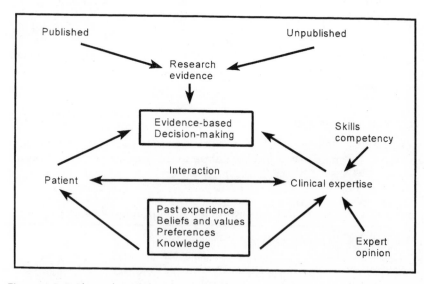

Figure 1.3 Evidence-based decision making.

it is appropriate for them. Once this has been decided, the options should be presented to patients in a way that enables them to be active participants in the decision-making process, if they choose to do so. Only then should a decision be reached as to the most appropriate treatment options.

This complex decision-making process, taking account of a range of evidence, informs the interaction between the healthcare professional and the patient as illustrated in Figure 1.3, adapted from the Chartered Society of Physiotherapy (1997).

Making decisions

As Stocking (1992) highlighted, evidence of an intervention's effectiveness, improving the health status of a patient, is only one aspect that might influence acceptance or rejection of that evidence. Other factors such as the time required to carry out the intervention, the ability to do so and the subsequent effect on costs, may all influence the perceived advantage of the evidence-based approach and its applicability. This issue is explored further in Chapter 2.

Revised definition

Having explored the definition of evidence-based medicine and reached a common understanding, it is helpful to rephrase it slightly. Substituting the term **practice** for **medicine**, and adding part of the following text which appeared in the original paper (Sackett et al, 1996), provides us with a clearer working definition:

> Evidence-based practice is the conscientious, explicit and judicious use of current best evidence in making decisions about the care of individual patients, integrating individual clinical expertise with the best available external clinical evidence from systematic research.

Steps to evidence-based practice

Evidence-based practice is reached by following a number of steps. These have been defined by Rosenberg and Donald, (1995):

1. Formulate a clear clinical question from a patient's problem.
2. Search the literature for relevant clinical articles.
3. Evaluate (critically appraise) the evidence for its validity and usefulness.
4. Implement useful findings in practice.

There is a fifth step that should be added to this, namely to evaluate the impact of change in practice. These steps are illustrated in Figure 1.4.

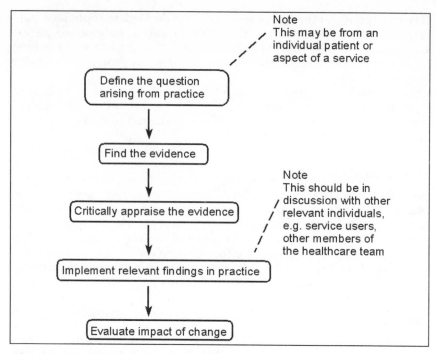

Figure 1.4 Steps to evidence-based practice.

Define the question arising from practice

As Figure 1.4 indicates, this may be about an individual patient or component of a service. How you define this **problem** will determine your approach and success at stage 2. Chapter 6 gives an example of how a clinical question needs to be broken down into its constituent parts if the search for evidence is to be successful. Some simple examples are presented here.

Example 1
You are part of a multiprofessional team working with adults with schizophrenia. You want to find out if cognitive rehabilitation approaches improve general function and mental state, and if they are acceptable to patients.

Intervention   = cognitive rehabilitation approaches
Outcome   = general function, mental state, Acceptability
Patient/problem = adult schizophrenia.

Example 2
You have been asked to investigate the potential benefits of setting up a hospital at home scheme for patients with terminal illnesses. These patients are currently cared for at the general hospital, because there is no hospice in the area.

Intervention   = hospital at home compared to in-patient care
Outcome   = benefit needs defining into specific outcomes, for
                   example, quality of life, function, morbidity,
                   mortality, cost
Patient/problem = terminal illness.

Example 3
You attend a multidisciplinary team meeting on the medical ward to discuss the management of acute stroke patients. It is suggested that reorganizing staff into a structured team to provide coordinated rehabilitation will improve the care of patients, reducing hospital stay and improving function and quality of life of patients. Before introducing a service change you decide to find out what evidence there is to support this move.

Intervention   = service – organized stroke care (you will need to
                   think of other ways of describing this and what it
                   might be compared to)
Outcome   = length of stay, function, quality of life
Patient/problem = acute stroke patients.

In defining the question, especially the outcomes to be reviewed, you will need to elicit what is important to the patient, not just your perspective as a practitioner.

Find the evidence

Chapter 6 covers this step in depth. It provides advice on where to find the research evidence, having developed your question into a search strategy, along with a review of the available resources. However, you are also reminded of the earlier discussion about different sources of evidence and should therefore not limit your information gathering to research evidence alone.

Critically appraise the evidence

Chapter 7 covers this step, as far as research evidence is concerned, and takes account of the range of methodologies that you might encounter. The checklists presented will help you to focus on the quality of articles, as well as answer questions about relevance and applicability. It is more difficult to apply the same systematic approach to the other types of evidence discussed. However, you need to balance their relative benefits, risks and influences on the anticipated outcomes.

Implement appropriate findings in practice

This step concentrates on what is done with the evidence. You may be faced with a relatively clear-cut decision informed by unambiguous research. This is more likely to be the case when the research from a number of studies has been synthesized for you in a systematic review or clinical guideline. However, it may also be vague, conflicting or absent. It is important to realize that not all searches for scientific evidence will result in definitive decisions, otherwise you will quickly become disillusioned. How to deal with uncertainty is discussed later in this chapter.

The relevant evidence needs to be discussed with the patient so that decisions about the most appropriate course of action can be taken. In doing so, the preferences of the patient are used to guide the final decision.

It is important at this stage to remember the influence of beliefs on outcome. Just as patients have beliefs, so too do practitioners. Your beliefs can impact on the implementation of findings in practice, so you need to ensure that your interpretation does not lead to errors in the application of the evidence. The process by which you reach a decision should be explicit so that it is possible to tell how the contributing sources of evidence have influenced the conclusions and recommendations made (Dowie, 1996). This has implications for record-keeping.

Implementation is about change to improve practice and patient outcomes. There has been a substantial amount of research investigating tools available to assist implementation, as well as specific approaches designed to change practitioner behaviour. These are discussed in Chapters 3 and 4. The use of clinical guidelines and clinical audit as tools for implementation are examined in Chapters 8 and 9.

Evaluate impact of change

It is important not to assume that by implementing the findings you will achieve the same results as the original research, or the desired outcome for the individual. Only through a process of evaluation will you be able to assess whether the decision has been successful or not. You can draw a similarity with your current practice, where you are evaluating the effect of your treatment on the patient and comparing this with your treatment goals. However, the difference is the evidence base to your treatment. Where change is on a large scale, not just an individual–practitioner encounter, such as change across a department or service, a more formal evaluation will be necessary.

How do you know if your practice is evidence-based?

Having a list of questions that you can ask yourself about each individual patient encounter is useful. The following set of questions is adapted from Greenhalgh (1996). Based on your assessment of the patient have you:

1. Identified the physical, psychological, social and any other problems?
2. Taken into account the patient's beliefs and preferences?
3. Competently performed a complete assessment to establish the presence of coexisting morbidity or pathology and determined how this might affect your conclusions?

4. Considered the interaction required with other members of the healthcare team and how this might affect treatment decisions?
5. Balanced the information gained from questions 1 to 4 to set priorities and agree goals with the patient?
6. Where necessary, sought relevant evidence from a variety of appropriate sources, such as clinical guidelines, systematic reviews and primary research to inform the treatment programme?
7. Assessed the quality, applicability and relevance of the evidence to this patient?
8. Presented the advantages and disadvantages of the different treatment options to the patient in a way that he or she can understand?
9. Incorporated the patient's preferences into the final recommendations and treatment programme, designed to achieve the goals set?
10. Reviewed the results of the treatment and compared them to the anticipated outcomes?

Multidisciplinary evidence-based practice

If evidence-based practice is to promote more clinically effective care then it must embrace all professional groups by providing a culture which is receptive and pluralistic in nature. If only one profession takes up an evidence-based approach then the risk is that power relationships and potential rivalry between professions will hinder patient care. The reality of healthcare is one in which several professions are involved at any time in providing care to individuals. Many examples of rehabilitation, such as head injury and drug addiction, are dependent on multiprofessional working. While there may be evidence to support the occupational therapists' role in rehabilitation, which they incorporate into their practice, how effective will this be without a similar approach from all those involved (speech and language therapists, clinical psychologists, nurses, etc.)?

What skills do you need to underpin evidence-based practice?

You may have already highlighted possible educational needs, such as searching for the evidence or critical appraisal skills. These are just two of the new skills you may need to develop or further enhance. You will have realized that evidence-based practice is about the process of change, which requires a range of skills, from those who will need to manage the change process to those who will need to implement it and affect personal change. If evidence-based practice is to fully involve service users then communication skills may need to be refined in order to elicit patients' preferences and expectations and involve them in the decision-making process. While you are probably already evaluating your practice on a day-to-day basis, you may need to consider how you can more systematically evaluate change across services or different healthcare professionals. Also, it is important that managers recognize their responsibility for creating a supportive environment in which this approach can be taken forward. These requirements for successful change are addressed throughout this book.

Dealing with uncertainty

Therapists do not have a long history of research, although there has been considerable growth since the 1970s. They are not alone. Even those professions which have a longer tradition in research, such as medicine, are experiencing similar difficulties in dealing with gaps in the evidence base for many areas of practice. A longer research tradition does not necessarily guarantee that interventions have a sufficient body of good-quality research on which to base decisions. As Appleby and colleagues (1995) have indicated, 'the current amount of evidence available is still limited to a small number of health care interventions, is of variable quality and can be difficult to obtain.'

The fact that many areas of healthcare do not have supporting evidence derived from research may be due to a number of factors (Appleby et al, 1995):

- Difficulties in designing studies
- Where interventions are already accepted practice, it may be considered unethical to withhold a potentially effective treatment in order to undertake clinical trials
- Existing research of poor quality
- Technology has moved ahead of research
- RCTs are not appropriate to all areas of healthcare
- While research may have taken account of clinical effectiveness, little attention has been paid to economic issues and therefore cost-effectiveness remains unaddressed
- Failure of research to be appropriately disseminated and made accessible.

The amount of available research will also be directly related to the amount of investment put into it. In addition, the ease with which the outcomes of an intervention can be measured will also influence the research undertaken. This may be particularly relevant to the therapy professions. Hope (1995) gave a good example of this when he compared the relative ease of measuring the outcome for an intervention aimed at correcting an acute medical problem, compared to the less clear-cut, longer term outcomes of interventions for people with chronic diseases.

So how do practitioners deal with uncertainty? It has been suggested that the human mind is malleable enough to allow the practitioner to adapt and become comfortable making decisions in the face of uncertainty, the so-called 'grey zones of clinical practice' (Naylor, 1995). Problems can occur, though, when personal opinion is equated with scientific evidence and when personal ignorance is confused with genuine scientific uncertainty (Naylor, 1995). The definition of evidence-based practice highlights the importance of clinical experience in informing the patient–healthcare professional encounter. Where scientific evidence is lacking, greater importance needs to be placed on clinical reasoning skills, drawing on experience and interpretation.

In some cases the scientific evidence may later be produced which affirms our personal opinions and leads some to ask, 'why do we need the research, when we knew all along we were right?' This brings us back to the need to appreciate that there are biases inherent within opinions. Research evidence, reinforcing practice, offers reassurance. There will also be instances when the scientific evidence calls into question previously opinion-based practice. This can be more difficult to accept and can lead some practitioners to dispute the evidence because it does not reinforce their beliefs. This is discussed in Chapter 4 which focuses on changing practitioner behaviour.

A patient may come to you who does not reflect any previous patient that you have seen. This uncertainty may be the trigger to seek further evidence. For many this means consulting another peer or expert (Turner and Whitfield, 1997). While a more senior colleague will be more experienced, it may be unclear how his or her knowledge base has developed. There is no guarantee that his or her advice will be based on the best available evidence, informed by research. However, in the absence of scientific evidence, it may be the best information available to guide clinical decisions. Where possible, though, clinical views should be complemented with a search for available scientific evidence.

Evidence-based policy

Generally, changes in policy are designed to improve health and change the way in which health services are funded and held accountable. To achieve this, changes will need to take account of the wider context of healthcare, encompassing the physical and social environment, as well as service provision (Gray, 1997). This is essential if evidence-based healthcare is to incorporate social services, public health, health promotion and education parameters as outlined at the beginning of this chapter.

Policy invariably has a political dimension. Decisions will be made not on evidence alone, but in response to the allocation of resources, and the values of politicians and their desire to carry favour with the electorate. However, with the introduction of the NHS R&D Strategy (Department of Health, 1991) the need to base decisions on evidence, was extended to policy-makers. As part of the Strategy there is a policy research pro-gramme (Department of Health, 1997a). This is directed at the health of the population as a whole. It includes studies of health and social well-being, lifestyle issues, health promotion and disease prevention, environmental factors and health service organization. Programmes of research are funded to inform policy. Areas such as skill mix and multidisciplinary working will be familiar to therapists. The outputs of such programmes may lead to the circulation of guidance and executive letters by the Department of Health in order to set direction and inform, or even dictate, healthcare management decisions.

Policy initiatives, such as clinical audit and primary care, are incorporated into the research programme. For example, research has been funded to document and analyse examples of clinical audit practice in clinical psychology, physiotherapy, occupational therapy and speech and language therapy, in order to provide guidelines for good practice. The shift to a primary care-led NHS has been a growth area in terms of policy initiatives and research funding (Department of Health, 1996, 1997a). The National Centre for Primary Care R&D is one centre funded by the policy research programme. In addition, the move to primary care-based commissioning is a major policy development in the White Paper *The New NHS: Modern, Dependable* (Department of Health, 1997b). While evidence to support these initiatives may not come directly from systematic research, they are often informed by past experience of previous organizational changes and common sense evaluations of the outcomes, although some are introduced with minimal evidence except that of opinion and ideology. They may then be exposed to systematic evaluation through policy-based research (Gray, 1997).

To encourage evidence-based social care there is a Centre for Evidence-Based Social Care, which has been set up to facilitate the translation of research results into service and practice developments. It also aims to improve the knowledge base of social work education and training.

Work is in progress to evaluate the impact of the reforms arising from the National Health Service and Community Care Act (1990), in areas such as services for older people and residential care. In pursuing this programme of research, consideration is given to the inter-agency collaboration required for the planning and delivery of social services, which includes a focus on joint commissioning, hospital discharge and continuing care, and primary care.

Similarities can be drawn between policy approaches and those of clinical practice. Invariably change has been introduced without a firm evidence base and the research then follows to try to substantiate the introduction. It would appear that many policy decisions are driven by fashion, pragmatism and idealism. This may be a result of problems regarding research time scales, the pressure to change policy and implementing policy decisions in practice. Also, there needs to be a shift from the biomedical model to a more social model (Hunter, 1997).

Through the commissioning process and resulting management decisions, policy decisions can have a direct bearing on clinical practice. For example, omitting certain drugs from the list from which general practitioners can choose, directly influences prescribing habits (Gray, 1997). Policy-makers should not pressurize practitioners to implement evidence-based practice without applying the same principles to their own decision-making.

Evidence-based commissioning/purchasing

Purchasing decisions tend to focus on:

- Particular groups of patients, such as elderly people
- Specific diseases, such as cancer
- Particular interventions, such as speech and language therapy, occupational therapy or physiotherapy.

A needs assessment informs these decisions and takes account of the prevalence of health problems within the population and the evidence that interventions provide more good than harm (Gray, 1997). With health services being provided in different sectors, such as primary or secondary care, independent or private sectors, purchasers will need to negotiate with a range of healthcare providers.

Those responsible for purchasing healthcare will have to make decisions that are guided by the policies and priorities of the Department of Health, the NHS Executive and other agencies, such as social services and education. At a more local level, consideration should be given to the public's needs, wishes and demands, the purchasing intentions of neighbouring areas, as well as pressure from providers to invest in particular services. Finally, purchasing decisions will need to take account of both clinical and cost-effectiveness issues. Therefore, decision-making needs to take account of conflicting perspectives (Appleby et al, 1995). Milne and Hicks (1996) recognized that the interests of commissioners cannot be served by evidence concerning effectiveness alone and needs to be supplemented with evidence concerning other dimensions of quality. Maxwell (1984, 1992) defined six dimensions of quality which, in addition to effectiveness, include accessibility, relevance, equity, acceptability and efficiency. These are explored further in relation to clinical effectiveness in Chapter 2.

There is already some concern that evidence-based practice will be misused by commissioners who elect to purchase only those treatments which have been shown to be effective (Polychronis et al, 1996; Maynard, 1997). There are major flaws in this approach, not least the fact that many areas have yet to be investigated, which should not be interpreted as ineffectiveness. This dogmatic use of evidence-based practice will ultimately deny patients treatments that they may have preferred and which were effective for them, which can only be viewed as unethical (Hope, 1995; Polychronis et al, 1996). Like practitioners, commissioners are faced with uncertainty in dealing with the evidence, as most effectiveness research focuses on interventions rather than patterns of care or the organization of services (Milne and Hicks, 1996). There are also likely to be similar education needs for those purchasing healthcare, such as developing information-searching skills and critical appraisal.

Like evidence-based practice, evidence-based commissioning provides opportunities. However, it may also lead down potentially dangerous decision routes as the next section outlines.

Rationing and evidence-based healthcare

Milne and Hicks (1996) suggested that the constraints of resource limitations, organizational change and professional defensiveness may lead commissioners to perpetuate long-standing 'must dos', such as reducing waiting lists. Also, that while services thought to be ineffective may be disinvested in, there is no guarantee that those shown to be effective will be increased. Rather than value for money, cost limitation becomes the focus.

Those purchasing services are well placed to use the various levers they have access to, at a policy level, such as research and development, education and training, contracting and audit, to influence change and facilitate opportunities (Milne and Hicks, 1996). This has the potential to:

- Facilitate training opportunities for staff to develop the skills necessary for evidence-based decision-making
- Influence the research agenda to fill identified gaps in the research evidence
- Facilitate the implementation of research in practice, but only if handled appropriately.

In the UK, the NHS continues to face resource constraints. This is unlikely to change due to increasing demands and expectations, the advances in new technologies and interventions, the ability to do more for those who previously went untreated and an ageing population (Hunter, 1996; Gray, 1997). Therefore, rationing is seen to be inevitable. In the absence of evidence, which applies to many areas of healthcare, and in view of the delays encountered of getting research into practice, there is little choice (Hunter, 1996). Until this gap is overcome, decisions will be based on what might at times appear to be arbitrary reasons.

Instead of talking about rationing, an evidence-based approach should promote discussions about prioritization which are based on sound information. This would make commissioners more accountable, and where they deviate from equitable and efficient healthcare provision they would need to be prepared to justify their course of action.

To fully inform healthcare commissioning decisions, evidence-based practice needs to encompass the range of methodologies already discussed, so that the focus is not simply on scientific efficacy, but also accounts for other factors such as acceptability, quality and cost. As Hunter (1996) argued, simply knowing that something is effective or not is not enough to inform policy decisions. It is important to know how effective an intervention is and to what degree of probability. Also, that other factors including the setting, history and values are incorporated into the decision-making process. If the decision-making process incorporates these factors then it should lead to more informed decisions about what to provide versus what to exclude in healthcare provision.

Evidence-based management

Once resources have been allocated, it is the responsibility of managers at the provider site to put them to work for the benefit of the population. This will include efforts to increase efficiency and quality, and to ensure that policy objectives are met (Gray, 1997). Managers are therefore directly influenced by both policy and purchasing decisions. In doing so they have responsibility to:

- Increase the provision of services/interventions that do more good than harm
- Stop services/interventions that do more harm than good
- Delay the introduction of new services/interventions with an unknown effect until they have been evaluated
- Promote change in practice by creating the right environment
- Work with professionals to ensure improvements in patient care and value-for-money services
- Promote research to fill identifiable gaps
- Ensure more coordinated efforts to decrease variation in practice, by facilitating and implementing agreed clinical policies (Gray, 1997).

Many of the essentials for good management and dealing with the change process are dealt with in other chapters in this book, in particular Chapter 3.

Balancing individual and population perspectives

'The policy and professional conflict between individual–patient ethic and population-health goals waxes and wanes and is often fought as a political battle' (Maynard, 1997). This conflict, in balancing the needs of individuals with those of the population, needs to be resolved if patient care is not to suffer as a consequence. Most practitioners focus on doing the best they can for individual patients. However, those who purchase healthcare do so on behalf of the populations for whom they have responsibility (Figure 1.5).

Potentially, evidence-based commissioning can be seen to be dictatorial, imposing a top-down dogma, which is insensitive to individual need (Milne and Hicks, 1996). Because of the population and service perspective of commissioners, they are well-placed to draw together all relevant stakeholders in reviewing the evidence and need for change. They will seek to maximize health gain for that population using their finite resources (Maynard, 1997).

Practitioners and managers also have responsibilities that extend beyond individual patients. Maynard (1997) argued that 'inefficient practice deprives other patients of care from which they could have benefited'. Focusing only on the individual may not acknowledge the benefits in terms of the future treatment of other patients within the

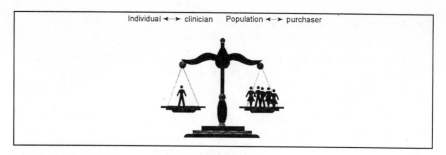

Individual ◄──► clinician   Population ◄──► purchaser

Figure 1.5 Balancing individual and population perspectives.

wider population (Maynard, 1997). Through evidence-based commissioning practitioners are expected to behave efficiently and ethically by taking account of both effects and costs in the care of patients.

So if evidence-based practice is about the individual ethic and evidence-based purchasing about the population ethic, how is common ground to be reached? Those purchasing healthcare need to change the focus of assessing health services on the basis of throughput and survival as the end points, to that of clinical outcome. This has been advocated in the government's *The New NHS: Modern, Dependable* (Department of Health, 1997b). Many conditions treated, especially by therapists, are of a chronic nature and should not be assessed in terms of mortality, but in quality of life. This means that commissioners need to focus more on valid outcome measures which take into account an individual's physical, social and psychological functioning when making their decisions. While these measures are used in clinical research and now more widely in clinical practice, greater consideration needs to be given to them by those purchasing healthcare.

As Gray and colleagues (1997) stressed, decisions usually require tradeoffs and will need to take account of individual as well as societal values.

Making it work in practice

Barriers will always exist in the face of challenges and change. It is important that these are acknowledged and understood if progress is to be made. Having an evidence-based approach should make you question your assumptions and beliefs, and in doing so encourage you to seek out evidence to answer questions. However, this requires time. It can easily be seen how the pressures of the workplace reinforce old habits, by inhibiting information-seeking and questioning behaviour. Some potential barriers, with which you may identify from personal experience, are presented below (Evidence-Based Medicine Working Group, 1992; Rosenberg and Donald, 1995; Sullivan and MacNaughton, 1996).

Barriers to evidence-based healthcare

- Time and effort
- Inappropriate infrastructure to support this approach to decision-making
- Gaps in the evidence
- Not enough high-quality evidence
- Available evidence is out of date or even wrong
- Lack of skills: critical appraisal, literature searching, use of information technology
- Perceived threat
- Lack of understanding of change process
- Economic constraints
- Relevant information available, but not easily accessible
- Information overload.

As in most cases, many of these potential and real barriers can be converted into opportunities, as illustrated below (Appleby et al, 1995; Rosenberg and Donald, 1995). It is important to take this positive perspective if progress is to be made.

Opportunities offered by evidence-based healthcare

- Improve patient care
- Close the gap between good clinical research and practice
- Promote self-directed learning and facilitate continuing professional development (CPD)
- Improve reading habits, information technology skills, literature searching and critical appraisal
- Promote teamwork
- Improve efficiency of practitioners
- Identify further research
- Stop activities known to be ineffective or even harmful
- Improve practitioners' understanding of research methods
- More effective use of resources
- Better information for patients, facilitating shared decision-making
- More informed approach to management, priority-setting and policy-making.

For those trying to take forwards evidence-based healthcare, it is important that barriers are identified and strategies developed for countering them, so that the opportunities can be realized. This is addressed throughout the book.

Summary

So what does an evidence-based approach have to offer? Ultimately it is designed to improve patient care based on informed decision-making. In doing so it also recognizes the need to cope with uncertainty and the gaps in the evidence. Therefore, it is important to have a clear understanding of what evidence-based practice is in order to avoid misinterpretation. It provides the opportunity to harness lifelong learning skills, developing a critical and systematic approach to incorporating evidence into decision-making. By decreasing the emphasis on opinion-led practice, it does not marginalize or negate experience derived from years of practice and what is learnt from educators and colleagues, but incorporates it into the decision-making process. These years of experience provide the insights into healthcare behaviours, along with skills in assessment and interpretation. Much of this cannot be gained from scientific evidence (Evidence-Based Medicine Working Group, 1992). Observations from practice also help to develop theories and ideas which can then be evaluated in a systematic way.

Practitioners, managers, policy-makers and purchasers need to develop strategies to deal with the explosion in information, seek out evidence and critically appraise it. In doing so, both old and new interventions will need to be evaluated if concerns about the rising costs of healthcare are to be managed effectively. An evidence-based approach also needs to shift the focus on performance from throughput to quality and outcomes.

Further reading

Gray, J. A. M. (1997). *Evidence-based Healthcare: How to Make Health Policy and Management Decisions*. Churchill Livingstone.
Sackett, D. L., Richardson, W. S., Rosenberg, W., et al. (1997). *Evidence-based Medicine. How to Practice and Teach* EBM. Churchill Livingstone.

References

Ad Hoc Working Group for Critical Appraisal of the Medical Literature (1987). Academia and clinic: a proposal for more informative abstracts of clinical articles. *Ann Intern Med*, **106**, 598–604.
Andrews, K. (1991). The limitations of randomised controlled trials in rehabilitation research. *Clin Rehabil*, **5**, 5–8.
Appleby, J., Walshe, K. and Ham, C. (1995). *Acting on the Evidence*. National Association of Health Authorities and Trusts.
Black, N. (1996). Why we need observational studies to evaluate the effectiveness of health care. *BMJ*, **312**, 1215–8.
Chartered Society of Physiotherapy (1997). *CSP Clinical Effectiveness Strategy*. Chartered Society of Physiotherapy.
Department of Health (1991). *Research for Health: A Research and Development Strategy for the NHS*. Department of Health.
Department of Health (1996). *Choice and Opportunity: Primary Care: The Future*. Stationery Office.

Department of Health (1997a). *Policy Research Programme. Providing a Knowledge Base for Health, Public Health and Social Care*. Department of Health.

Department of Health (1997b). *The New NHS: Modern, Dependable*. Stationery Office. .

Dowie, J. (1996). 'Evidence-based', 'cost-effective' and 'preference-driven' medicine: decision analysis based medical decision making is the pre-requisite. *J Health Serv Res Policy*, **1**(2), 104–13.

Evidence-Based Medicine Working Group (1992). Evidence-Based Medicine. A New Approach to Teaching the Practice of Medicine. *JAMA*, **268**(17), 2420–5.

Gladman, J. R. F. (1991). Some solutions to problems of the randomised controlled trial in rehabilitation research. *Clin Rehabil*, **5**, 9–13.

Gray, J. A. M. (1997). *Evidence-based Healthcare: How to Make Health Policy and Management Decisions*. Churchill Livingstone.

Gray, J. A. M., Haynes, R. B., Sackett, D. L., et al. (1997). Transferring evidence from research into practice: 3. Developing evidence-based clinical policy. *Evidence Based Medicine*, **2**(2), 36–8.

Greenhalgh, T. (1996). "Is my practice evidence-based"? *BMJ*, **313**, 656–7.

Haynes, R. B., Sackett, D. L., Gray, J. A. M., et al. (1996). Transferring evidence from research into practice: 1. The role of clinical care research evidence in clinical decisions. *Evidence Based Medicine*, **1**(7), 196–8.

Hicks, N. (1997). Evidence-based health care. *Bandolier*, **4**(39), 8.

Hope, T. (1995). Evidence based medicine and ethics. *J Med Ethics*, **21**, 259–60.

Hunter, D. (1997). *Science Based Policy Making in the UK: The Case of the NHS*. 2nd International Conference Scientific Basis of Health Services, Amsterdam.

Hunter, D. J. (1996). Rationing and evidence-based medicine. *J Clin Eval*, **2**(1), 5–8.

Maxwell, R. J. (1984). Quality assessment in health. *BMJ*, **288**, 1470–2.

Maxwell, R. J. (1992). Dimensions of quality revisited: from thought to action. *Qual Health Care*, **1**, 171–7.

Maynard, A. (1997). Evidence-based medicine: an incomplete method for informing treatment choices. *Lancet*, **349**, 126–8.

Milne, R. and Hicks, N. (1996). Evidence-based purchasing. *Evidence Based Medicine*, **1**(4), 101–2.

Moore, A., McQuay, H. and Gray, J. A. M. (eds). (1995). Evidence-based everything. *Bandolier*, **1**(12), 1.

Mulrow, C. D. (1994). Rationale for systematic reviews. *BMJ*, **309**, 597–9.

Mulrow, C. D. and Oxman, A. D. (eds). (1997). Glossary. Cochrane Collaboration Handbook [updated September 1997]. In *The Cochrane Library* [database on disk and CDROM]. The Cochrane Collaboration. Update Software, 1997, issue 4.

National Health Service and Community Care Act 1990 (*c. 19*). (1990). HMSO.

Naylor, C. D. (1995). Grey zones of clinical practice: some links to evidence based medicine. *Lancet*, **345**, 840–2.

NHS Centre for Reviews and Dissemination (1996). *Undertaking Systematic Reviews of Research on Effectiveness: CRD Guidelines for those carrying out or commissioning reviews*. CRD Report 4. University of York.

Polychronis, A., Miles, A. and Bentley, P. (1996). The protagonists of 'evidence-based medicine': arrogant, seductive and controversial. *J Clin Eval*, **2**(1), 9–12.

Rosenberg, W. and Donald, A. (1995). Evidence based medicine: an approach to clinical problem solving. *BMJ*, **310**, 1122–6.

Sackett, D. L., Rosenberg, W. M. C., Gray, J. A. M., et al. (1996). Evidence-based medicine: what it is and what it isn't. *BMJ*, **312**, 71–2.

Stocking, B. (1992). Promoting change in clinical care. *Qual Health Care*, **1**, 56–60.

Sullivan, F. M. and MacNaughton, R. J. (1996). Evidence in consultations: interpreted and individualised. *Lancet*, **348**, 941–3.

Turner, P. and Whitfield, T. W. A. (1997). Physiotherapists' use of evidence based practice: a cross-national study. *Physiother Res Int*, **2**(1), 17–29.

2

Clinical effectiveness: another perspective to evidence-based healthcare

Judy Mead

What is clinical effectiveness?

Clinical effectiveness is defined as:

> The extent to which specific clinical interventions, when deployed in the field for a particular patient or population, do what they are intended to do – i.e. maintain and improve health and secure the greatest possible health gain from the available resources. (NHSE, 1996a)

Clinical effectiveness is about ensuring that clinical interventions are based on the best available evidence, as described in the previous chapter. Effectiveness, however, is about **applying** such interventions within real-life conditions. Research evidence, in particular, may have been derived from interventions carried out in ideal conditions. This will demonstrate their **efficacy**, but will not necessarily, if applied in the usual conditions of healthcare, be **effective** (Working Group for the Director of Research and Development of the NHS Management Executive, 1993). Conditions, including the environment, organizational systems and patient characteristics, need to be weighed up, alongside information about the treatment's efficacy. A decision can then be made about the applicability and likelihood for health gain of that intervention in those circumstances. The nearer these components can be to the ideal, the more confident patients and health professionals can be of achieving a beneficial outcome. While patient characteristics cannot be changed, other than in a long-term health promotional sense, the environment and organizational systems can be altered, providing greater potential for ensuring consistently high quality. Clinical effectiveness, therefore, is achieved by using interventions that are known to work, and embedding these within an environment and systems that are of the highest possible quality.

Another way of describing clinical effectiveness is presented by Graham (1996) as the six Rs: 'the **right** person, doing the **right** thing, the **right** way, in the **right** place, at the **right** time, with the **right** result'. In other words:

- Was the **person** delivering the care competent to do so? Did he or she have the necessary skills and knowledge to assess the patient's problem and deal with it? Could someone with less skill and experience have been as effective? Did the person take proper account of the patient's preferences and experience? Did the practitioner enable the patient to feel a partner in his or her own care and decision-making?
- Was the right **thing** done? Was there evidence to support the effectiveness of the intervention? Did the patient agree to the intervention?
- Was the intervention used in the right **way**? This might be a question of skills and competence, or it might be about meeting national standards or guidelines for that particular process. Was the process acceptable to the patient? Was the dignity and privacy of the patient maintained?
- Was the intervention given in the most appropriate **place**? Could the patient have been treated at home rather than making a long journey to hospital? Did the patient understand the need to travel, in order to receive the intervention from a clinician who was familiar with his or her rare condition, and where specialist equipment was available?
- Was the intervention given at the right **time**? Would it have been more effective if the patient had not been on the waiting list for six months? Was the patient given adequate time to consider the implications of the intervention before making a decision whether or not to go ahead? Was the intervention given at a time when carers were able to support the patient during it or afterwards?
- Did the intervention achieve the right **result**? Did it do what it was intended to do (NHSE, 1996a)?

Linking clinical effectiveness and quality

Before the term **clinical effectiveness** became a buzzword, **quality** was a term used more commonly. Six dimensions of healthcare quality were described by Maxwell (1984, 1992) as: access; relevance to need; effectiveness; equity; acceptability; and efficiency.

Some of these dimensions, for example effectiveness, access and acceptability, overlap the six Rs. Others, such as efficiency and relevance to need, are given greater emphasis by Maxwell, whose dimensions incorporate a population, as well as an individual, perspective to health-care. A population perspective highlights the importance of providing the most good for the population as a whole, within limited resources. This theme has already been considered in the previous chapter, and is echoed in the NHSE (1996a) definition of clinical effectiveness, which emphasizes the need to 'secure the greatest possible health gain from the available resources', and is discussed further in this chapter.

You might feel daunted at the prospect of all these components of quality needing to be considered for the achievement of clinical effectiveness. However, there should be anticipation as well. If a **patient's experience of care** is to be of the highest quality, to which most health professionals will want to aspire, they all warrant close attention, alongside the need to base practice on the best available evidence, as described in the previous chapter.

Often, the terms **clinical effectiveness** and **evidence-based practice** are used interchangeably. However, this book differentiates between the terms. Clinical effectiveness encompasses evidence-based practice, but places it within the context of wider environmental and organizational aspects of healthcare systems (Chartered Society of Physiotherapy, 1997). This acknowledges the importance of considering evidence-based clinical interventions not in isolation, but taking account of a range of dimensions of quality in the application of such interventions, for individuals and for populations. By doing so, it will be possible to provide the most effective quality experience and the most health gain for the population. The importance of the wider healthcare environment in achieving this is reflected in the previous chapter's discussion of evidence-based healthcare, of which practice is one element.

The history of clinical effectiveness

Clinical effectiveness was an initiative promoted by the UK government of the day, around 1991. Some of the underlying issues which may have been behind the government's thinking are discussed later in this chapter. The initiatives were promoted through the National Health Service Management Executive (NHSME), later the National Health Service Executive (NHSE), when a national Research and Development (R&D) programme was set up under the direction of Sir Michael Peckham. It had five key functions (Department of Health, 1991).

- To ascertain the knowledge that NHS decision-makers need
- To ensure that knowledge was produced
- To make the knowledge available to decision-makers
- To promote the implementation of R&D findings
- To promote an evaluative culture.

The initiative was perhaps an acknowledgement that, in the past, some research had been funded that had limited impact on developing new knowledge about the most effective healthcare, either through inappropriate topic selection, or through inadequate use of the research in practice. The emphasis changed to ensure that priorities were based on research need, rather than influenced by vested research interests, and new information was generated that could be implemented in practice (Haines and Jones, 1994).

In 1993, the first Executive Letter about clinical effectiveness, EL(93)115 (NHSME, 1993), was sent to purchasers and trust chief executives. It exhorted, 'the NHSME wishes to see better use made of research-based evidence about clinical effectiveness'. In 1994, a similar letter, EL(94)74 (NHSE, 1994), stated 'improving the effectiveness of clinical services must be a constant aim'. A requirement to develop action plans to achieve this aim was made in the *Priorities and Planning Guidance, 1995/96* (PPG) (NHSE, 1995a). The high priority attached to clinical effectiveness has continued to be in evidence. For example, one of six medium-term priorities in the PPG for 1997/98 specifies 'improve the clinical and cost effectiveness of services throughout the NHS and thereby secure the greatest health gain from the resources available, through supporting R&D and formulating decisions on the basis of appropriate evidence about clinical effectiveness.'(NHSE 1996b, 1997). A change of government has not lessened the emphasis. *The New NHS: Modern, Dependable* (Department of Health, 1997) also commits the service to ensuring clinically-effective and cost-effective care.

From an early stage (NHSE, 1994), emphasis was placed on the importance of:

- Partnerships between purchasers and health professionals
- Using clinical guidelines as a way of involving patients
- Using clinical audit and professional education as tools to ensure the implementation of evidence of effectiveness and changing of professional practice.

All of these are discussed within this book.

There were also requests (NHSE, 1996c) not to invest in the use of new health technologies or screening programmes prior to recognized assessments of their effectiveness.

In 1996, the NHS published more extensive guidance on clinical effectiveness in *Promoting Clinical Effectiveness: A Framework for Action In and Through the NHS* (NHSE, 1996a). This described three main themes:

- Inform (making evidence of effectiveness accessible)
- Change (using well-founded information to encourage changes to services)
- Monitor (assessing changes in services to ensure that they have resulted in improvement).

These are discussed in later chapters. Some describe different aspects of the same theme, but each is required to achieve the complexities of clinical effectiveness. For example, strategies for achieving change are discussed in a number of chapters, with an organizational change management approach taken in Chapter 3, examples that are supported by research evidence in Chapter 4 and the role of patients in facilitating change in Chapter 5.

The document *Promoting Clinical Effectiveness: A Framework for Action In and Through the NHS* (NHSE, 1996a) acknowledges clinical effectiveness as a complex process which involves clinicians, managers and patients themselves. It states, 'Everyone has a part to play in bringing clinical evidence, judgement and experience together to make rational decisions about changing healthcare practices'.

Clinical effectiveness: whose responsibility?

Interest in making health services more effective appears to be a theme common to many countries. In the UK, a number of stakeholders will each have a view about their own, and others', responsibilities. Common to all, however, should be a commitment to:

- Achieving the greatest health benefit for the population for whom they have responsibility
- Reducing inappropriate variations in practice
- Ensuring value for money
- Involving individual patients and the population in decisions about their personal healthcare and the wider needs of the population, respectively.

The stakeholders will include:

- Politicians, who are accountable to the general public, yet whose motivation may be popularity with voters and, ultimately, re-electability
- Consumers of healthcare, who are also payers, through the taxation system, and, for some, payers for private care
- Purchasers and commissioners of healthcare who, in the UK, need to get the best value from finite resources for the population as a whole
- Providers of healthcare (health professionals), whose businesses or jobs rely on an agreement with funders to deliver services. They are likely to have an inherent sense of professional responsibility to do good rather than harm, and to provide high standards of care (Maxwell, 1984).

For all the stakeholders, whatever their underlying motivation, there is something to be gained (a common element of 'added value') in the achievement of increasingly clinically effective healthcare, for example through evidence-based policy-making, management and patient choice, as discussed in the previous chapter.

Politicians

'Ministers have been quick to promote evidence-based medicine as the principle means by which to square the circle of growing demands on the

NHS on the one hand and finite public resources on the other. It allows them to argue that a knowledge based NHS will ration only that which is of proven ineffectiveness as distinct from ad hoc, arbitrary rationing' (Hunter, 1996). Was the clinical effectiveness programme set up as rationing, by another name? Was it about cost cutting?

There was a political expectation that it would be possible to stop health professionals doing things that did not work, and ensure that they only did those things which were known to do good. The logic appeared to be that this would lead to cost reductions in otherwise tight, finite resource limits. However, the reality is that it cannot be assumed that effective interventions are cheaper than ineffective ones, or that health professionals will easily change their practice to reflect the knowledge base, or that the knowledge base is complete. Such forecasts may therefore have been somewhat optimistic, not least because of the relatively limited amount of reliable research evidence available on what is effective or ineffective. Just because interventions are of unproven effectiveness, it cannot be assumed that they are ineffective.

At the same time, huge sums of taxpayers' money have been invested in the national R&D programme, including funding for the UK Cochrane Centre and the Centre for Reviews and Dissemination in York (both described in Chapter 6). This was a significant commitment to the generation of new knowledge, both through new primary research and the synthesis of existing research.

The political expectations may have been higher in relation to cost reductions than is realistically deliverable. The task of demonstrating value for money is therefore great. Will politicians lose patience if the clinical effectiveness programme fails to reduce costs and improve health?

Consumers of healthcare

The Patient's Charter (NHSE, 1995b), provides patients with a right to be involved in decision-making. The Charter states 'You (the patient) have a right to be given a clear explanation of any treatment proposed, including any risks and any alternatives, before you decide whether you will agree to the treatment'. Patients, therefore, require good information about the effectiveness of interventions and their relative benefits and risks, so that they can make an informed choice and give properly informed consent. Patients will become increasingly skilled in assessing the research evidence for themselves through critical appraisal (Burls and Milne, 1996) and in using the Internet as a source of information. They will then be able to make more rational decisions about the services they prefer.

In 1985, a study by Greenfield et al found that a group of patients with peptic ulcer disease who were coached to improve their information-seeking skills in order to interact more effectively with their physician had better outcomes related to physical well-being than those who were not coached. Duff et al (1996) defined the prerequisites for patients to be involved in decision making. Access to information, an understanding of the options open to them and the confidence to participate in decision-making were determined as among the key factors.

These studies suggest that the empowerment of consumers, through access to information and partnership with health professionals, may have an as yet untapped potential for improving health. Consumers also have a right to be involved in policy- and decision-making about the needs of the whole population nationally and locally, through the ballot box and through local fora respectively. *The New NHS: Modern, Dependable* (Department of Health, 1997), goes some way to acknowledging this in its promise to explore ways of securing informed public and expert involvement in decisions about local services that are planned. These issues are discussed in greater detail in Chapter 5.

Patients need to see themselves as partners in their care. This can only be achieved if professionals acknowledge this partnership and facilitate it. The attitude 'I'm the professional, therefore I must know best' may be declining, but it needs to be eradicated. Therapists of sensitivity, who maintain an awareness of the wider issues in healthcare, will want to adapt their behaviour over time and reap the reward of knowing that they are meeting patients' needs more effectively.

Purchasers and professionals need to come to terms with the fact that increasingly patients may be at least as well-informed as they are, or demand to be so. Indeed, instances where patients feel they have not been given adequate information or been inadequately involved in their own or their children's care, may lead to litigation. A sensible professional will readily enter into a partnership with a patient to enhance his or her understanding where necessary, while acknowledging and putting to good use the very real contribution that patients bring in relation to their own experience and values.

Projects to enhance information available to patients about their care have included the MIDIRS series of leaflets (MIDIRS and the NHS Centre for Reviews and Dissemination, 1996). These aim to give women who are pregnant a view of the available research findings about specific aspects of pregnancy and childbirth, for example ultrasound scans in early pregnancy and positions for labour and delivery. The leaflets are produced in pairs, one designed for users and the other to support professionals, which includes more detailed information and references. The use of the leaflets therefore guides both women and professionals through decisions involved in childbirth.

Consumers have responsibilities as well as rights. On an individual level, their responsibilities include:

- The avoidance of waste through missed appointments or inappropriate call-outs
- Taking responsibility for their own healthcare, where appropriate.

Issues about consumers' responsibilities for leading a healthy lifestyle are complex and not a subject dealt with in this book. Perhaps it is sufficient to highlight the ethical dilemmas of, on the one hand, the consumer as a payer of healthcare through taxes, arguing for freedom and liberty to smoke cigarettes, eat certain foods and take no exercise, all likely to lead to health and social costs, and even premature death. On the other hand, there is the responsibility an individual has to ensure that resources are available for all, particularly those with diseases that are not preventable, or for those whose low level of income makes a healthy lifestyle difficult.

Purchasers and commissioners

Purchasers and commissioners make decisions about buying healthcare for the population they serve, using taxpayers' money. They therefore have a moral and ethical obligation to get the best deal for their population, with the resources at their disposal. They need to consider the provision of the most effective interventions for promoting good health, for regaining or maximizing health following disease or disability, and providing care for long-term needs.

They have to face the same challenge as many professionals in acknowledging a great deal of healthcare for which there is little, if any, good research-based evidence of effectiveness. Those who want to reduce the costs of healthcare may use the lack of research-based evidence as a reason to cut healthcare expenditure in these areas. However, there may be evidence for some treatments simply because a lot of money was put into research in those areas, for example by drug companies. Equally, some outcomes are more easily quantifiable than others. The difficulty of measuring outcomes of interventions for people with chronic diseases, coupled with a purchasing policy of relying on high-quality randomized clinical trials for evidence of effectiveness, could act against the interests of those with chronic disabilities, causing ethical concerns (Hope, 1995). While there may be difficulties in researching areas, where less clear-cut and longer term outcomes are required, other ways need to be found of eliciting evidence of effectiveness for these patients. Greater use could be made of asking patients in a systematic way about their experience of care. Failure to address this issue could lead to a bias, to purchasing only those treatments where there is good research-based evidence of effectiveness (Hope, 1995).

To implement evidence-based purchasing, as described in the previous chapter, purchasers need to develop appropriate skills. This might be in the critical appraisal of research literature, or the management of change, or communication and facilitation skills. Purchasers need to be on a level playing field with professionals, to be able to resist the likelihood of being influenced by vested interest. In a study conducted in South West Thames region (Littlejohns et al, 1996), where clinicians and purchasers met together in small workshop sessions to explore their relationship, as part of a process to agree patterns of care based on research evidence of proven effectiveness, the beliefs and assumptions that purchasers and professionals made about each other were elicited. Professionals felt that purchasers were:

- Heavily influenced by political and financial considerations
- A lay body that could not understand the clinical issues

- Unlikely to heed advice given by professionals, or would seek advice from those professionals who would tell them what they wanted to hear.

Purchasers, in turn, felt that professionals were:

- Likely to give advice that was belief- rather than knowledge-based
- Biased to their own service and professional body aspirations.

A range of inducements was agreed as acceptable to purchasers and providers:

- Educational interventions aimed at increasing research awareness among purchasers and providers
- Incentives through performance management agreements with the NHSE, and the use of quality assurance schemes such as clinical audit. This was later reinforced in a report, *Acting on the Evidence: Progress in the NHS* (Walshe and Ham, 1997), in which the authors recommended the need for stronger and more effective performance management mechanisms to ensure the effective implementation of clinical effectiveness by trusts and health authorities
- Incorporating evidence-based clinical guidelines into contracts and monitoring through clinical audit.

The use of service reviews, involving those providing care as well as purchasing, provides a tool for promoting clinical effectiveness (Walshe and Ham, 1997). A combination of a systematic approach to exploring the evidence base, with the involvement of all stakeholders in the existing service, appeared to have greater potential for bringing about change. However, this needs to take place in an environment that is prepared to consider the best **available** evidence, rather than dismissing services that are not supported by evidence from high-quality randomized controlled trials, as discussed earlier.

Purchasers have a key role to play in developments in practice. Interventions that are proven to be ineffective should not be purchased. Where there is unproven effectiveness, purchasers may want to introduce such services as part of a properly designed and ethically approved trial, or at least delay their spread until such trials are undertaken (NHSE, 1996c). However, innovations that have been shown to be effective should be promoted enthusiastically.

Twenty years ago, Archie Cochrane, whose work inspired the mission of the Cochrane Collaboration, to provide better information about what works and what does not in healthcare, identified the need to base healthcare decisions on the degree of health gain and cost-effectiveness. He wrote, 'there will also be limitations on the present administrative freedoms. Allocations of funds and facilities are nearly always based on the opinions of senior consultants, but, more and more, requests for additional facilities will have to be based on detailed argument with hard evidence as to the gain to be expected from the patient's angle and the cost. Few can possibly object to this' (Cochrane, 1977). Such a statement is just as relevant in an environment of commissioning healthcare today.

Professionals

As professionals, therapists and others have a number of responsibilities:

- A duty of care to their patients, which overarches all other responsibilities
- To aspire to the raising of standards (Maxwell, 1984)
- To use funding, whether paid indirectly through tax or directly for private care, appropriately and efficiently, minimizing waste and maximizing benefit
- To maintain their ability to work safely and competently (Chartered Society of Physiotherapy, 1995; College of Occupational Therapists, 1995; Royal College of Speech and Language Therapists, 1996).

A culture that reflects and aspires to meet these responsibilities can be fostered through continuing professional development (CPD). Its role in facilitating the incorporation of research evidence into practice is described in Chapter 4, and its importance as a tool for the successful implementation of clinical guidelines is described in Chapter 8.

Through the use of appropriate CPD programmes, professionals can be more confident of meeting their responsibility to continue to work safely and competently. The adoption of all the practical components of this book should ensure that therapists are:

- Providing care to patients based on the best available evidence
- Delivering care within high quality systems
- Providing a good experience of care for patients
- Creating opportunities for patients and professionals to work in partnership.

The achievement of these should reduce the likelihood of a professional being subject to litigation. So clinical effectiveness can be seen to be an effective tool for risk management as well as for quality improvement.

Service managers, as professionals alongside clinicians, also have a responsibility to facilitate clinical effectiveness. Chapter 3 highlights the importance of organizational change and the factors that need to be in place to achieve this, among which management involvement is key. Walshe and Ham (1997), for example, reported that it was difficult to start a meaningful dialogue about clinical effectiveness without good relationships between clinicians and managers.

Professional bodies

Most professional bodies consider a key function to be the setting and monitoring of professional standards. The monitoring process achieves another key role: that of protecting the public from incompetent practitioners, or practitioners whose behaviour to patients is inappropriate. Professional bodies will, therefore, want to support their members in delivering clinically effective services to patients. They need to ensure that national standards, including nationally developed clinical guidelines, are based on the best available evidence and that the CPD programmes they promote facilitate the provision of more effective and higher quality services for patients. With the revision of the Professions Supplementary to Medicine Act of 1960 (Department of Health et al, 1997), it seems likely that the government and professional bodies will act in partnership to assure themselves of professionals' continuing competence to practice. The monitoring and measuring of the effectiveness of individuals' CPD activities will be a key component in this process.

Haines and Jones (1994) state 'Professional associations have an important role to play in ensuring that research based information is included in educational activities and clinical guidelines'. The NHSE also sees a significant role for professional bodies in the development and monitoring of clinical guidelines. 'The development, publication and maintenance of guidelines remains the responsibility of the appropriate professional body ...' (Mann, 1996). Funding does not necessarily follow such statements, however, so the development of clinical guidelines is likely to be limited to high priority topics (see Chapter 8). Increasingly, professional bodies are working in collaboration with each other, and with service users, in order to ensure that the guidelines are more meaningful to practice.

In partnership with training establishments, professional bodies also need to ensure that pre-qualifying programmes take account of the available evidence in the scope of clinical practice that is taught. A culture of evidence-based and clinically effective practice needs to be developed in students in a way that will influence their lifelong learning and is seen as integral to being a professional.

Clinical effectiveness: efficiency and ethics

In another far-sighted comment, Cochrane (1977) wrote, 'I cannot agree that colleagues, however distinguished, intelligent and hardworking, and who obviously believe they are doing good should have a blank cheque ... without bothering to measure the benefit and cost of what they are doing'. Such a strong statement, addressed to the medical profession, about the ethics of doing good but also weighing benefits against costs to ensure value for money, was rare at the time that Cochrane wrote it. Today, it is a less surprising statement, but remains one that is all too easily overlooked or ignored. Cost–benefit analysis is still rarely carried out as part of the research process. However, it should be considered in making a decision about whether the investment in an intervention for an individual or as part of a wider service is going to provide value for money. For example, in a study of supervised fitness walking in patients with osteoarthritis of the knee (Kovar et al, 1992), one of the outcomes showed that following the programme, patients could walk at least 10 per cent and up to 27 per cent further in a six-minute test of walking distance. However, the programme involved 24 90-minute walking and education sessions over an eight-week period, led by a physical therapist. The question, therefore, in deciding whether or not to use that research evidence in practice, is: was there enough **benefit** to patients to warrant the **cost** of providing the intervention, or the **cost to the patients** in terms of time? Other consumer issues that emerge from this paper are discussed in Chapter 5.

Culyer, in 1992, questioned not just the wasted resources of doing something inefficiently or ineffectively for particular patients, but the ethics of what that means in terms of **potentially wasted benefit to others**. Inefficiency and ineffectiveness can therefore be a double whammy. Available funds fail to benefit the patients being targeted and there are also wasted opportunities for others who could have benefited.

Therapists have as great an ethical responsibility as other health professionals to manage their resources efficiently. For example, there is a duty of care to patients on waiting lists as well as to those undergoing treatment. There is therefore a need to ensure that those patients who do receive treatment are those likely to benefit, otherwise the resource is wasted. Other considerations might include:

- How long does the programme last? Are reviews of progress adequate or sufficiently frequent?
- Could the length of visits or programmes be reduced if more experienced staff were available, or if more training were given to those currently available?
- Are referrals appropriate? Has there been a dialogue with referrers to agree criteria for referral, including options other than therapy for patients with genuine needs, but for whom therapy is used as a placebo?

Therapists must be committed to achieving an effective service, but also one which is responsive. The provision of such a service goes back to elements of the six Rs: the right person; doing the right thing; the right way; in the right place; at the right time; with the right result.

Another ethical issue in healthcare, highlighted in *The New NHS: Modern, Dependable* (Department of Health, 1997), is the wide variation in practice across the country. The ethical concerns are about equity of care across populations. How many people working in the health service have said 'If I'm going to have an accident (or a stroke, or heart attack), I hope I'm taken to x hospital and not y'. Therapists know, by talking to colleagues working in other hospitals, that stroke rehabilitation, for example, appears to be more successful in some places than others. This might be due to a range of factors, including variations in the quality of care of other professional groups, or resources available to employ staff. However, lack of research evidence is still hampering knowledge of the efficacy of different therapy-led approaches or interventions. Some variations may, therefore, be due to the use of different approaches by therapists. There is strong evidence, however, that stroke care provided by a specialist multidisciplinary team saves lives, compared to stroke patients being managed routinely in medical wards (Stroke Trialists' Collaboration, 1997). Indeed, the evidence shows that where organized stroke care is in place, one extra life can be saved for every 16 patients admitted, compared to non-organized care. It is distressing, therefore, that organized stroke care may still not be uniformly available in the UK.

As more systematic reviews and well developed clinical guidelines are written, clinicians will be able to access clearer information about what works (is effective) and what does not. Such evidence still needs to be applied, however, through one or more of the many models for change management described in this book. If successfully implemented, this may be one factor in successfully reducing variations in healthcare across the country in the future.

Systems to ensure clinical effectiveness

Healthcare organizations, including those basing their services on the best available evidence of effectiveness, must also examine the processes, or systems, within which those services are being delivered. Are the systems efficient? Is there room for improvement?

Business process re-engineering

Business process re-engineering (BPR) is a tool which, when applied successfully, can have a dramatic effect on efficiency, on reducing costs and, most importantly, on improving the experience of patients. It focuses on processes rather than functional boundaries, and considers why and what should be done, before how (Clarke and Poulter, 1997). At Derbyshire Royal Infirmary, the introduction of nurses initiating X-rays at triage in an accident and emergency setting speeded up the identification of fractures. At Leicester Royal Infirmary patients received test results in 36 minutes instead of 79 hours (Clarke and Poulter, 1997). The authors identified the following key characteristics of successful BPR in three NHS trusts:

- The vision and purpose were clear
- Multidisciplinary teams were involved
- Real control existed over the processes
- There was a real focus on the patient
- Communications were well managed.

Are there examples in therapy services where re-engineering would benefit patients? Why are therapy services normally provided on a Monday-to-Friday basis? Do patients not occupy beds, or suffer pain or disability at weekends? If the evidence were to show that treatment on a daily basis was more effective than intermittent days, could services be re-engineered? An example of introducing a seven-day therapy service for orthopaedic patients is described in Chapter 3. Reviewing skill mix is another form of re-engineering, reorganizing services where necessary to ensure patients are treated by those whose skills most closely match their needs.

Re-engineering is a complex process where organizations need to adopt a style of listening and discussion, rather than telling (Clarke and Poulter, 1997). The rewards can be great, thinking afresh about systems that will truly meet the needs of patients rather than the needs of staff or the organization.

Benchmarking

Benchmarking provides another opportunity to look at effectiveness and efficiency with an ethical dimension. If common data, using agreed definitions, were to be collected across the country and showed wide variations, for example in lengths of hospital stay for patients having a knee replacement, you would want to know why. If your hospital had longer stays than others, you would want to see if there was anything you could learn from the experience of those achieving shorter stays, to improve your own local systems and experience for patients. Were your interventions different to those of other services? Which were based on the best available evidence? If the interventions given were broadly similar to those given by other services, what else was different? Were patients seen more or less frequently? How much information was given to patients? Were the knowledge and skills of the rehabilitation team different between the best and worst performing services? There would need to be good clinical data on the in-patient episode, as well as on outcomes. For example, it would be important to ascertain levels of functional ability on discharge, and the proportion of readmissions, to ensure that a short length of stay was not compromised by worse outcomes. The bottom line is what can you learn from those who appear to provide better services to patients, in order to provide better services to your own patients.

Using data to measure performance has been a backbone of performance management for many years. Until recently, the measuring of performance has been in relation to efficiency and economy, but not effectiveness, even when effectiveness has been a commitment at policy level (Walshe and Ham, 1997). Examples are cited by the authors of surgeons performing ineffective procedures for those who have been on waiting lists longest, in order to reduce them, when the surgeons could have been performing effective procedures on other patients. The Secretary of State for Health, however, in *A New NHS: Modern, Dependable* (Department of Health, 1997) acknowledges a history of perverse incentives 'which got in the way of providing efficient, effective, high quality services'. The document promises better measures which will 'assess the NHS against the things which count most for patients'. Greater emphasis will be placed in future on **clinically relevant** performance indicators and the use of outcome measures, to provide more meaningful indications of whether or not health services are meeting the needs of those who use them.

Integrated care pathways

Integrated care pathways (ICPs) are structured multidisciplinary care plans which detail essential steps in the care of patients with a specific clinical problem (Campbell et al, 1998). In other words, they describe the anticipated course of a patient's passage through the health system for that particular clinical situation. Discussions across professions and across departments will identify a step-by-step approach to the process: what should happen, by whom and when. This provides an opportunity, not dissimilar to process re-engineering, to review existing processes and to think afresh about solutions to known problems. For example, the writing of an integrated care pathway for stroke patients in the Bassetlaw Hospital and Community Services NHS Trust led to support staff being able to accompany occupational therapists on home assessments, freeing up the time of another occupational therapist who would otherwise have attended. The involvement of speech and language therapists in the training of dysphagia link nurses, allowed an increase in the dysphagia service from five to seven days a week (Moody et al, 1995). Increasingly, pathways consider the evidence base for the interventions being considered. So pathways that are not only based on the best available evidence, but which are also embedded within efficient and effective systems, provide a **gold standard** for ensuring clinical effectiveness. The benefits of ICPs (adapted from Ellis, 1997) can be described as:

- Less record-keeping: a multidisciplinary chart needs only to be initialled if care for a particular patient is in accordance with the pathway
- Structured information: the structured information on the chart, including information on variances from the pathway, facilitates the review and updating of the pathway
- Better-informed patients: the patient has access to the pathway (usually kept at the end of the bed), and is therefore informed of what events can be expected
- Educational: an information tool for new as well as established staff, which improves multidisciplinary and clinician–patient communication
- Increased consistency in care: reducing inappropriate variations in practice
- Reduction of risk: by having an agreed, thought-through, evidence-based process for care, easily accessible to staff and patients alike, leading to a better-educated team, likely to perform better
- Reduced costs: this might be achieved, for example by reducing length of stay, by designing optimum processes that are achieved consistently rather than being dependent on the right staff members being available, e.g. the consultant's ward round.

There is a further potential benefit from the use of pathways, as they are in themselves tools for audit. Record-keeping systems are established which detect variations from the pathway (exception reporting). These can then be discussed by the team to identify whether this was caused by a systems failure, which may indicate the need for the system to be modified, or a person failure in not adhering to the pathway, which might imply a training or other staff development need.

Summary

Clinical effectiveness has been described in this chapter as the application of evidence-based practice in a multifaceted and complex environment. Interventions must be based on the best evidence available, whether this is drawn from research evidence, from clinical expertise or from patients. Evidence-based interventions need to take account of patient choice, reflecting patients' experiences and patients' values. Costs, risks and benefits of specific interventions need to be considered. Further dimensions, of having effective and efficient systems within which to deliver care equitably, which provide patients with a good experience at the time they can most benefit, with appropriately skilled people, making best use of available resources, complete the complex picture that can ensure that clinically effective services are achieved.

References

Burls, A. and Milne, R. (1996). Evaluating the evidence: an introduction. *J Clin Effect*, **1**(2), 59–62.

Campbell, H., Hotchkiss, R., Bradshaw, N., et al. (1998). Integrated care pathways. *BMJ*, **316**, 133–7.

Chartered Society of Physiotherapy (1995). *Rules of Professional Conduct*. Chartered Society of Physiotherapy.

Chartered Society of Physiotherapy (1997). *Clinical Effectiveness Strategy*. Chartered Society of Physiotherapy.

Clarke, S. and Poulter, J. (1997). Business process re-engineering: a framework for improving healthcare. *Br J Healthcare Comput Inf Management*, **14**(9), 16–17.

Cochrane, A. L. (1977) *Effectiveness and Efficiency: Random Reflections on Health Services*. British Medical Journal and The Nuffield Provincial Hospitals Trust.

College of Occupational Therapists (1995). *Code of Ethics and Professional Conduct for Occupational Therapists*. College of Occupational Therapists.

Culyer, A. J. (1992). The morality of efficiency in healthcare – some uncomfortable implications. *Health Economics*, **1**, 7–18.

Department of Health (1991). *Research for Health: A Research and Development Strategy for the NHS*. Department of Health.

Department of Health (1997). *The New NHS: Modern, Dependable*. Stationery Office.

Department of Health, Scottish Office Department of Health, Welsh Office, Department of Health and Social Services for Northern Ireland (1997). *The Health Professions Bill: Draft Specification*. Department of Health.

Duff, L. A., Kelson, M., Marriott, S., et al. (1996) Involving patients and users of services in quality improvement: what are the benefits? *J Clin Effect*, **1**(2), 63–7.

Ellis, B. W. (1997). Integrated care pathways: implications for clinical risk management. *Healthcare Risk Rep*, **May**, 13–15.

Graham, G. (1996). Clinically effective medicine in a rational health service. *Health Director*, **June**, 11–12.

Greenfield, S., Kaplan, S. H. and Ware, J. E. (1985). Expanding patient involvement in care: effect on patient outcomes. *Ann Intern Med*, **102**, 520.

Haines, A. and Jones, R. (1994). Implementing findings of research. *BMJ*, **308**, 1488–92.

Hope, T. (1995). Evidence-based medicine and ethics. *J Med Ethics*, **21**, 259–60.

Hunter, D. (1996). Evidence-based medicine is no panacea. *Health Director*, **June**, 12.

Kovar, P. A., Allegrante, J. P., MacKenzie, C. R., et al. (1992). Supervised fitness walking in patients with osteoarthritis of the knee. *Ann Intern Med*, **116**(7), 529–34.

Littlejohns, P., Dumelow, C. and Griffiths, S. (1996). Implementing a national clinical effectiveness policy: developing relationships between purchasers and clinicians. *J Clin Effect*, **1**(4), 124–8.

Mann, T. (1996). *Clinical Guidelines: Using Clinical Guidelines to Improve Patient Care Within the NHS*. NHS Executive.

Maxwell, R. J. (1984). Quality assessment in health. *BMJ*, **288**, 1470–2.

Maxwell, R. J. (1992). Dimensions of quality revisited: from thought to action. *Qual Health Care*, **1**, 171–7.

MIDIRS and the NHS Centre for Reviews and Dissemination (1996). *Evidence Based Informed Choice in Maternity Care*. Informed Choice.

Moody, L. Rowland, K., Fairclough, F., et al. (1995). Different strokes. *Health Serv J*, **9 May**, 26–7.

NHS Executive (1994). EL(94)74. *Improving the Effectiveness of the NHS*. Department of Health.

NHS Executive (1995a). *Priorities and Planning Guidance, 1995/96*. Department of Health.

NHS Executive (1995b). *The Patient's Charter and You*. Department of Health.

NHS Executive (1996a). *Promoting Clinical Effectiveness: A Framework for Action In and Through the NHS*. Department of Health.

NHS Executive (1996b). *Priorities and Planning Guidance, 1996/97*. Department of Health.

NHS Executive (1996c). EL(96)110. *Improving the Effectiveness of Clinical Services*. Department of Health.

NHS Executive (1997). *Priorities and Planning Guidance, 1997/98*. Department of Health.

NHS Management Executive (1993). EL(93)115. *Improving Clinical Effectiveness*. Department of Health.

Royal College of Speech and Language Therapists (1996). *Communicating Quality: Professional Standards for Speech and Language Therapists*. Royal College of Speech and Language Therapists.

Stroke Trialists' Collaboration (1997). Specialist multidisciplinary team (stroke unit) care for stroke inpatients. In *Stroke Module of the Cochrane Database of Systematic Reviews* [updated 01 December 1997] (C. Warlow, J. Van Gijn, P. Sandercock, et al., eds) Available in The Cochrane Library [database on disk and CDROM]. The Cochrane Collaboration, issue 1. Oxford: Update Software, 1998 [updated quarterly].

Walshe, K. and Ham, C. (1997). *Acting on the Evidence: Progress in the NHS*. NHS Confederation.

Working Group for the Director of Research and Development of the NHS Management Executive (1993). What do we mean by appropriate health care? *Qual Health Care*, **2**, 117–23.

Facilitating Change

Making evidence-based healthcare happen requires change. This might be required at any number of levels, such as at an organizational, service, department or individual level. These are likely to be interdependent. The successful management of change requires commitment, understanding and a supportive environment, along with a recognition of the need for change. Everyone will carry some degree of responsibility for this change process, but the level of action will vary.

There are recognized strategies for managing and influencing change at both an organizational and an individual level. These are presented to provide you with a range of approaches which can be implemented depending on individual circumstances. Throughout, the need to recognize barriers to change in order to be successful is stressed.

The increasingly important role of consumers in influencing change in healthcare is explored. This is a significant move if partnerships in decision-making are to be encouraged. It is an evolving area in which therapists will want to engage.

3
Change management

Jane Keep

> Life at its best is a flowing, changing process in which nothing is
> fixed... (Rogers, 1967)

As every healthcare professional will have experienced, life in healthcare
organizations during the 1990s has become increasingly more complex,
diverse and fragmented, with the twenty-first century bringing a myriad
of new influences all having a changing effect on the workplace. Most
recently, *The New NHS, Modern, Dependable* sets out far-reaching
changes for the whole of healthcare and those working within it. 'The
NHS cannot stand still. It needs to modernize if it is to meet patients'
aspirations for up-to-date, quicker, more responsive services'
(Department of Health, 1997).

Service reconfigurations, the influence of medical technology, and
indeed the impact of evidence-based healthcare leave professionals with
many complicated puzzles to wade through. Creating stability within
change presents a major challenge for those working within healthcare
teams. Change itself requires both team and personal reflection in order
to understand where, if any, working practices could be improved. Good
change management practice includes the need for training or
development in addition to reviewing and improving communication.

Many changes are forced upon a team or individual by external factors,
and certainly an essential part of practising and managing within the
health service is to learn to predict and respond positively and
optimistically to external factors. Internal factors also precipitate change,
although cause and effect are hard to elicit. How many external factors
have caused internal factors? Many, most likely. Internal factors can be
from within teams or within individuals themselves and could, for
example, be around the decision to train a team further in a particular
skill, or an individual's wish to learn more about a particular practice.
Each is part of a change process. Professionals and managers are faced
with the challenge of being proactive in terms of planning the future and
more effective in the provision of services or treatments. This is often

coupled with the challenge to be reactive, faced with many, often bureaucratic, organizational policy agendas or continuous cost pressures.

Evidence-based healthcare is itself a change perspective that brings with it the need to integrate research into day-to-day practice. For a reflective practitioner, who may regularly reflect upon his or her own practice or think critically in order to ensure that the best and most effective clinical practice is being undertaken, the gap is not such a chasm. However, for an action-orientated practitioner, who works diligently using well-established practices, going from one patient to the next, leaving little time for reflection or critical thought, this gap can be vast. Some level of evidence-based or, at a minimum, reflective practice, is at the forefront of future organizational and individual practice, not just for practitioners but for a whole range of other professions and management practitioners within healthcare. Understanding the need to develop and practise tasks in a reflective and evaluative manner places the need for those involved in change, which is most health care practitioners, to rely increasingly on integrating research into practice. Measuring achievement, evaluating effectiveness and sharing good practice allows reflection to take place.

Key features of successful change management

Consider the following case study and the lessons learnt as an example of successful change management.

Case study

A working group was formed within a healthcare organization to look at the use of speech and language therapy assistants. The group consisted of the assistants themselves, therapists and managers. The group broke their remit down into tasks and goals, starting by looking at the scope of the role, training needs and how, or whether, to move to a set of competencies for the assistants, linked to improved pay scales.

Consideration at the early part of this project was given to the needs and aspirations of the assistants in full consultation with them. Immediate needs and longer term career aspirations were considered. Many issues were discussed by using a form of SWOT (strengths, weaknesses, opportunities, threats) analysis so that both positive and negative aspects were discussed openly.

The end result was to engage the assistants in new, quite complex, clinical programmes with appropriate training. Looking at these posts as stepping stones for their future careers, and the steps required, proved effective for the assistants, the speech and language therapy service and the patients.

Lessons learnt

- Using those involved in the change to work as part of the working group led to full participation and involvement

- Understanding the needs from both the therapists' and assistants' perspectives led to greater openness, trust and collaboration
- Unpacking the concept, for example in this case the scope of the role of an assistant at an early stage, enabled a firm foundation to be built upon for the duration of the project
- The general acceptance of all those involved of both how the change had been undertaken and the overall principle and goals of the change itself helped commitment and prioritization of those involved
- Reviewing and monitoring of the project throughout its duration encouraged continuous improvement.

Change problems and keys to success

When thinking about change and the types of issues that teams or individuals face, it is useful to note both the problems and the keys to success. Many teams tackling change programmes suffer from a lack of :

- Focus
- Understanding of priorities
- Vision or direction for the future
- Project or action planning
- Participation from team members.

Problems can include the legacies of previous failed attempts at change, which have been carried out too narrowly without thinking about the future consequences. In addition, there is a temptation to attempt quick fixes rather than longer term approaches. **Change fatigue** can quickly set in. Indeed, teams and individuals that fail to manage change effectively can run the risk of wasted resources, difficulties with service delivery, or demoralization of the teams and individuals involved.

Successful change, therefore, lies in:

- Discussion
- Participation
- Reflection
- Adequate planning of resources, such as time.

Working together pulls the **change force** quicker in the new direction. By encouraging open minds to challenge and critique, the ability to be flexible and to change working practices for the future can be sustained. Understanding the nature of change itself, as a key process, provides an excellent foundation for assessing and implementing change. Successful change is possible, but there is much that can be done to improve current change practice.

Of particular importance is the fact that there are many *cookbook* approaches to managing and implementing change. Airport and railway bookstands are full of them! It is useful to have an insight into some of these, including the use of case histories to highlight specific points. However, *cookbook* approaches in the 1990s are not always appropriate without local contextualization and environmental workplace sensitivity.

This means having a true understanding of how work is carried out in your workplace and why it is carried out that way. Each framework or model for change will then need tailoring to local needs in order to ensure that the change is carried out, appropriate to the local working environment.

There is an important question to raise at this stage for all those becoming involved in change. Can change management, in any circumstance, be standardized, or is it too diverse to measure and therefore evaluate? Many would say that it is too diverse, and that separating cause and effect within any change programme is not an easy task. However, well-planned, monitored and evaluated change can work towards integrating evidence in practice.

What is change management?

'Over-hyped, under-implemented: past its sell-by date' (Bulletpoint, 1994). It has become an overused cliché, that the only certainty in life is uncertainty, and that the agenda for professionals and managers is one of continuous change. In a chapter such as this, it is not possible to outline all change writers and perspectives, but there are many basic concepts and ideas that can be highlighted.

Starting with the basics, change can be defined as 'the act or an instance of becoming different', 'an alteration or modification', 'a new experience; variety', 'the substitution of one thing for another; an exchange' (Coulson et al, 1991). To manage is defined by the same authors as 'organize; regulate; be in charge of', 'gain influence with or maintain control over', with management defined as 'the process or an instance of managing or being managed'. Placing these two concepts together, change management can be seen as a process of managing an act of becoming different, or the organization of an alteration or modification. There are many variations on this theme, such as Marshall's (1995), who states 'change is not change but rather a rearrangement or development of what was happening before'.

Types of change

Much is written about change and its variations, so what types of change are there? Any number of distinctions can be made such as those shown in Table 3.1.

Triggers to change

So what triggers change? There are many triggers such as those discussed earlier in this chapter. These can be clustered in ways such as the following (Salaman, 1992):

• **Working practices**: implementing evidence-based healthcare; acces-

Table 3.1 Types of change

Small scale e.g. the addition of security locks to an office window	**Large scale** e.g. the implementation of the new NHS patient numbering system
Radical e.g. a hospital move from an old site to new premises on a different site	**Incremental** e.g. a gradual change in the skill mix of a particular team, monitored and evaluated during an ongoing time scale
Content e.g. pressure sore care	**Process** e.g. a communication system such as team briefing, versus **Structural** e.g. the implementation of a new team-based organizational structure
Individual e.g. learning a new interpersonal skill such as negotiation	**Team** e.g. creating a new set of quality standards against a particular set of work practices

sing educational resources; improving complaints procedures; establishing standards
- **Management practices**: new organizational structures; systems of communication such as team briefing; new information systems
- **Organizational or wider healthcare practices**: evidence-based practice; clinical effectiveness; implementing Research and Development (R & D) infrastructures; efficiency drives.

Effecting change

In order to implement changes, each will require a different approach, dependent upon:

- The context/environment within which change takes place
- Time scales
- Available resources
- The speed of the change
- The individuals or teams to be involved
- Their preferences, skills or knowledge about the change itself.

Each change thus brings with it a set of challenges and hurdles, or bridges to cross, prior to its successful completion.

In addition, there are many possible change-hindering behaviours such as:

- Lack of cohesion or clarity
- Rigid or unrealistic views
- The punishment of risk-taking
- Professional tribalism or competitiveness
- Defence and blame routines that can be found within working groups.

Looking more positively, there are as many change-helping behaviours such as:

- The ability to focus
- Individual or team flexibility
- Personal or organizational commitment
- Good listening and other collaborative practices
- Good communication systems
- Monitoring or evaluation of change so as to understand at any one time where the change has reached.

All of these can be developed over time, and can be sensitive to the working environment, or the needs of the team and the individual in achieving change.

Guiding principles

In supporting the need for promoting and facilitating positive change behaviours, Burnes (1992) cites guiding principles for undergoing change which can generally be accepted as good practice:

- **Strategy**: how the programme relates to future objectives/priorities and how it affects the operation and structure of the (healthcare) team
- **Phasing the change**: creating the recognition of the need for change, making it happen, and consolidation
- **Involvement**: participation of those involved to enhance the quality of the change itself with wider perspectives, and the cooperation of those affected
- **Informed choices** and commitment: generating valid information and providing informed choice for those involved
- **Effect behaviour change**: facilitating and enabling those involved to change their behaviour to varying degrees
- **Culture change**: this invariably takes place following the above, although it may be an end in itself.

In taking a case study to outline this we can see how each of these guiding principles can work towards a positive change process.

Case study

- **Strategy.** This was around the need for patients, particularly routine orthopaedic post-operative patients, to receive the same treatment regime, regardless of the day of the week of their operation. A review was undertaken of current practice, and how seven-day weeks could be implemented so that a strategy could be developed.
- **Phasing the change.** The problem itself required recognition and action plans during the change process, with time for consolidation and review.
- **Involvement.** Consequences of any change were mapped at this stage with all parties who would be affected. Cooperation and collaboration was required from all involved: managers, all clinical professionals, and those who the change was looking to help, the patients.
- **Informed choices.** In order for any change strategy to be written and action

plans to be developed, information relating to the past service, and issues facing patients who were not able to receive a seven-day service was collated. Practice in other parts of the country was investigated, so that informed decisions could be made about the future of the service.

- **Effect behaviour change.** The roles, responsibilities, skill mix and working times of all involved in the proposed change were reviewed. Looking at current and potential future working practices, in addition to any individual needs and issues to be accounted for, were important factors if behaviour change was to take place. Working with the professionals providing the service, enabling them to review their own services and behaviour, was key at this stage.
- **Culture change.** Monitor and review mechanisms were placed in situ whilst the change was undertaken. Reviewing everyday working practices, communication and participation throughout showed that culture change had taken place in addition to the overall structural changes to the service provided.

Lessons learnt

When looking at change from a team perspective there is much that can be learnt, particularly with reflection, and of course hindsight! Writers on change would suggest that in some form or another, creating the right conditions within which the change should take place is an important component of successful change. Within the early stages of any change process, consideration would include:

- Ensuring some form of (change) needs analysis
- Looking at stakeholders (e.g. patients, other professionals, carers) who may be involved in the process, and who should be involved or informed
- The development of clear objectives
- Planning adequate resources and time for the change to take place
- Commencing monitoring mechanisms to continuously keep tabs on where the change is heading, not least leading to an evaluation at the end to see whether the proposed change has actually taken place.

In support of this early preparation, one of the most important features is to have a goal or blueprint for the future to aim for. All plans will have hurdles to cross whether these are obvious at the beginning, or emerge during change. However, having a strong future goal is important.

Guiding principles in relation to multiprofessional teams

A case study relating to managing change in implementing clinical effectiveness within multiprofessional teams highlights some interesting issues.

Case study

In a community NHS trust, enhancing clinical effectiveness via self-directed, multiprofessional teams was seen to be the way forward in delivering services. A variety of discussions had taken place as to what clinical effectiveness within a self-directed team might look like. To this end, a pilot was commenced.

A literature search was first undertaken to find cases of best practice (and poor practice), using research and case study literature. In addition, networking took place with similarly placed teams in other healthcare organizations. As a result, it was felt that a pilot could serve to gain information for a future framework or model for enhancing clinical effectiveness within a multiprofessional, self-directed team. Specific literature was limited, although there were some models of practice gained from fellow professionals outside the trust.

A clinical practice facilitator was assigned to work with the team, and a project plan was drawn up. Consultation with the team itself at this point was fairly rushed, and despite in-depth discussions no clear blueprint for the future had been formulated either within the team or within the organization itself. Resources and legitimate time had, however, been given in support of this project. A series of planning and teamworking events then took place, looking at the team's present state and towards the future in relation to the clinical services currently provided. The team completed the early stages of this project feeling energized, with many ideas and a set of objectives which it was to focus on in the coming months. However, although there had been positive initial evaluation from the team, later follow-up and subsequent meetings with the team revealed otherwise.

Some infighting had taken place following the initial project phase, whereby jockeying for individual status, or rank between senior members of the team, had become an issue. In addition, searching questions around clinical and professional practice had been raised between team members when looking at clinical standards. This subsequently required further facilitation and support, but their organization had, at this point, felt that it had given the time and support it had initially estimated was required and therefore left the team to get on with it. Worse than this, many of the ideas and objectives, once back in the workplace, were much harder to get off the ground than the team had envisaged.

Although there was broad support from the organization, certain support functions, such as adequate information technology or data collection systems, were not ready or able to support changes in their work practice. The organization's management team had evidently not thought through the real impact that improving clinical effectiveness could have on other parts of the organization or, indeed, the meaning of self-directed, multiprofessional teamwork. It was distinctly uncomfortable with being challenged or asked for advice on matters it had not considered previous to this pilot project.

The longer term outcome showed much demoralization within the team, with many of its initial ideas and objectives never being fulfilled. Although this was revisited at a later stage, the ground lost during this pilot phase was never really recovered. Subsequent review and evaluation showed that the organization had not been ready for this team to change practices.

Lessons learnt

- When undertaking change of any sort at team or service level, the rest of the organization needs to be involved right from the start
- Organizations need to fully understand their own ability to fulfil initial commitments to specific teams or projects, in addition to undertaking some kind of future scenario mapping issues to identify the implications that they will have for the organization
- There is always more support required than planned for, particularly in relation to time and other resources. Things always take longer to get

off the ground than envisaged, particularly when levels of patient care cannot be allowed to drop while change is undertaken
- Morale and motivation are very delicate in times of change, and require ongoing nurturing and support
- Even if you do look around at good practice elsewhere, or use litera- ture, you must take heed of the messages they give, both good and bad. Their experiences are strong indicators for learning from what has gone before
- While there is literature about clinical effectiveness (quoted in other chapters), and good practice and advice on teams, such as Belbin (1981), Margerison and McCann (1990) or Anderson et al (1990), it is important to note that there is also a need to use the much wider body of knowledge and practice related to change management. Teams and individuals will need to look at processes, and specific jobs and role boundaries, mapping the over- and underlaps within the change, even if deemed to be small.

The other useful learning point from the case studies presented so far (of which there are many similar examples) is that individuals require the ability to display a key range of skills such as resilience, openness and facilitation. All of these can be developed at early stages of any change process, with a little foresight and forward planning.

The individual and change

Turning things in the light, seeing a different impression as I do so, sometimes glimpsing many layers underpinning one surface repre- sentation. No one image is the only truth, or the only plausible account although some may feel more authentic, consistent with a person's values being more chosen than imposed. (Marshall, 1995)

We are all individuals, and see things from different perspectives, even if we can describe them in exactly the same way as the person standing next to us. Change requires an acceptance of this, as each part of the prism is our own, albeit we may think we all share that vision.

Covey (1989) describes personal change as 'creating a relationship between something you understand and something new'. The manage- ment of change requires those working within change to have high levels of skills and knowledge in relation to the change process, in addition to being able to manage themselves through these same change processes. Managing people in changing situations is not easy, neither is undergoing any personal change.

The anthropologist Vann Gennep (1960) discusses the **rites of passage** as transitions and rituals taking place throughout our lifetimes. These can be mirrored within organizational or team life cycles and within individuals who undergo change. Recognized change pathways can include phases of shock, anxiety, depression, denial, acceptance and reordering, although arguably not all changes will follow certain patterns or cycles, or will follow each of these states. Lao Tzu is quoted as saying 'Knowing others is wisdom, knowing yourself is superior wisdom' (Lindenfield, 1992). This sends a strong message to all those involved in change, relating to the need to understand yourself, perhaps via your own reflections and learning from previous changes, so that you can understand others while undergoing or implementing change.

People require many things when going through change, including recognition, advancement, interest and overall security. If change threatens any or all of these, the change can become difficult, if not impossible, to pursue with the individual or team involved. Certainly, when coercion or threats are used to implement change, it may seem as though change has taken place initially, but this is often superficial, and underpinning this change in attitude or behaviour, has probably not taken place at all.

Some may argue that it is unethical to require deep personal change to take place, and question the right we have to change individual behaviour or attitudes. However, whether this is legitimate or not, the purpose of change needs to be made clear to all who will be affected, and communication and participation are paramount.

Put another way, individual changes in working habits, skills and practice can bring with them a number of personal consequences or personal reactions. For the healthcare team this brings both personal and team consequences or reactions, thus there is a need to remain resilient, open and flexible. Added to this, tribalism from professional and managerial boundaries, or from one profession to another, or even within professions, brings with it the barriers of language or jargon in understanding each others' worlds, leading to possible disharmony or lack of collaborative working. Consider the following case study.

Case study

A newly appointed therapy manager, who managed a number of small groups of therapists, wished to influence a change in working practice for one of these groups. The manager had tried discussing with the group members what they might do about the particular issues relating to improved working practice, brainstorming their own solutions to the problems. Relations between all parties at this point were superficially amicable, although it seemed likely that any pressure on the relationship could mean a sudden breakdown.

Having tried via seemingly congenial discussions to undertake various changes in practice, with little or slow response, the manager decided that she should take a more directive approach, in that this small group should be told what it was to do. To this end, some attempts at coercion took place. Much resistance followed in various forms, for example excuses for not attending various meetings, or no contribution at all when present. Mainly, resistance was covert and difficult to detect, although the overall outcome was that the change itself was not evident. The distance between the manager and the group grew, and more particularly one or two members became withdrawn. The changes had the potential to raise the profile of the group and standards of care overall, but would put pressure on the amount of personal flexibility in working practices and in where (which site) the work took place.

This continued for some months. The manager had further discussions and head scratching sessions with other managers. A further view was sought from a number of individuals throughout the organization who were not directly involved or affected by the change, and who had a more distant relationship with both the manager and the team concerned.

Interesting discussions followed. It appeared that neither party had put themselves into the other's shoes, looking at the other's perspective. The change was felt to be inevitable and although the manager was seen as the primary change manager, the group was particularly under pressure from others, for example consumers of the service, to change. No-one had, up to this point, thought about or discussed what the motivators for this particular change would be, or what personal fears or aspirations were present at that time. Consequently, any action by the manager to change the way in which the practitioners practised had not taken into full consideration their individual or personal needs and expectations at that particular time.

Lessons learnt

- Although this may sound less complicated than one might have envisaged, these types of misunderstandings or misperceptions often cause the most problems when managing change
- Issues such as timing, motivation, unrealistic goals and, above all, remembering each individual, result in people facing change differently
- Individuals matter, and sensitivity to this is important
- Individual or personal expectations and aspirations differ markedly when investigated
- If individuals reflected more regularly about themselves while undergoing change, they might be able to see these other perspectives.

Managing change

There is a wealth of frameworks and tools relating to change management, some of which are described in the following sections. Some deal with specific tasks within change management and some relate to the overall process of change itself.

The quality, depth and scientific nature of the information and data relating to the frameworks and techniques differ markedly. The range includes:

- Handbooks
- Audio and video cassettes
- Popular press
- Sharing practice
- Research-based approaches found in peer-reviewed journals or academic papers and research reports.

To the novice, an element of terror could set in when faced with such a vast quantity of information and literature available! However, this also lends itself to a greater opportunity for exploration and choice, finding those practices that intuitively feel more approachable, or those that relate more readily to your working environment. Additionally, there is a body of change literature specifically pertaining to healthcare, with some being UK-focused.

One particularly important point to note relates to the contextualization or environmental specificity of these frameworks. Organizations and people are much more complex than organizational change practice and research imply. Thus, solutions to problems are also more difficult to grasp than implied. It is not possible to take a *cookbook* approach to managing change. However, it is useful to look through the cookbook first to understand some of the basic principles of managing change. Good cooks often use basic, foundational knowledge, e.g. making a white sauce, upon which their own innovation and creativity builds more interesting options for meals, e.g. making a soufflé. Good change practitioners would almost certainly do the same in understanding the basic change issues (communication, participation and involvement) and moving to more complex techniques (organizational analysis and diagnosis). All of this would be undertaken with the added knowledge of how they personally function and cope with change, as well as trying to understand how others function and cope with change too.

Change frameworks

You are already familiar with one framework for change, illustrated in Figure 1.4. in Chapter 1. Building on this, there are other, similar frameworks outlined here.

Change management is not all doom and gloom, and indeed many of the principles of perceived good change management offer much hope and opportunity towards getting things right, or having the desired effect.

Lewin's model of change

Kurt Lewin (1958) is one of the early social scientists who developed a model of change. Indeed, many other models use his model as their foundation. Lewin's model has been used for decades in organizations undergoing change. The model is divided into three stages:

- **Unfreezing:** where some impetus or issue, for example dissatisfaction (e.g. Patient's Charter), would drive the team or individual to the need to unfreeze current attitudes and behaviours. For example, a complaint from a patient may require an investigation into a particular practice. The outcomes of this determine that a change is necessary. The investigation itself serves as the first move towards changing, that is, questioning and analysing

- **Changing:** includes exploration of new ways of working, exchanging previous practices and approaches for new behaviours and approaches. Continuing the example, analysis leads to the need to search for new solutions, new ways of working, different approaches which would be more satisfactory to the patient(s). A pilot, or testing one or two new ways of working, could follow. A new approach is then found, and taken as the best way forward for a particular practice
- **Refreezing:** establishment of a new, stable equilibrium, reinforcing and institutionalizing practice. Continuing the example, this new working practice is continued, monitored and evaluated and soon becomes the norm for this team/individual.

While this provides a useful overview in relation to managing change, it appears to give the impression that this is a one-off process, and that refreezing actually takes place. In many organizations, change is continuous, thus leaving the refreezing phase slightly more flexible or open-ended in preparation for a continuous change approach. In the above case, continued monitoring or evaluation will inevitably lead to more subtle or evolutionary changes.

Beckhard and Harris' model

An adapted and extended model of Beckhard and Harris (1987) usefully outlines five stages:

- **Phase 1: looking at the need for change**. Why change a practice, when it has been used for the past 10 years quite satisfactorily: what is the impetus?
- **Phase 2: defining the future state.** So what might the new future practice look like? What should it achieve?
- **Phase 3: undertaking some form of present state analysis**. What exactly happens now?
- **Phase 4: devising an implementation plan.** What do we need to do to change and to implement the new practice?
- **Phase 5: undertaking the implementation while 'business as usual' takes place.** The new practice is implemented among other day-to-day working practices.

Looking at each of these phases in more detail:

Phase 1
The need for change can at times be undertaken by looking only at the tip of the iceberg, and thus missing the crux or core of the issue as to why change. Icebergs highlight explicit and overt systems and processes, structures and espoused working practices at the tip, those which are visible to the human eye. Much pre-change analysis is only undertaken at this visible level, missing a myriad of highly qualitative information which is implicit, covert and includes attitudes, behaviours and actual working practices, below the tip of the iceberg.

Phase 2

Defining the desired future state is often unrealistic or peripheral. For instance, before encouraging individuals to work in an empowered way, the term 'empowerment' itself requires breaking down into behaviours, skills, attitudes and knowledge, in addition to looking at all specific workplace practices that may be required to support such an initiative. The other important factor here is planning for contingencies or consequences of the change itself. No change takes place without some need for review, further planning or adaptation. Contingency measures should be built in at an early stage, and risks should be planned for.

Phase 3

Undertaking some form of organizational audit or present state analysis must be taken from both sides of the iceberg: the tip and that which is less obvious. The more exploration at this stage, the better the understanding and planning for the future change will become.

Phases 4 and 5

Looking at both getting from here to there and managing during the transition state, managing the implementation is paramount. Organizations cannot rely on professionals enacting change as a night job while expecting them to work at full capacity during their day jobs. This requires legitimizing the change project or task itself, which includes estimations of time and other resources to support this.

One further point to note is to make links to the wide body of literature surrounding project management and project management techniques. Project management offers an excellent change management framework which assumes that there is a beginning and end to the change itself. Within this there are a variety of key phases that can be undertaken using project management methodologies. Linking project management to change can place a rigorous framework of implementation, monitoring and evaluation. Much can be learnt from other professions outside the public sector, such as the building trade, from surveyors or from engineering, in the way that resource utilization is forecast and costed.

Change management tools and techniques

Taking the frameworks a step further, there is a range of tools and techniques that can be utilized.

Content, process and control

Buchanan and Boddy (1992) provide a useful outline to three agendas in any change situation which require effective management, namely content, process and control. These can be summarized as:

Content (this can be the technical or clinical tasks):

- Setting the content agenda, ensuring that all aspects of the change are addressed, including task, structure, people and technology issues
- Clarifying the task objectives and benefits: gathering ideas, developing clear objectives, setting measurable targets, testing for reality and acceptability
- Developing solutions to support the objective: ensuring that a coherent strategy is formulated which supports the change
- Bringing in the change and handing it on: phasing and timing the change implementation, ensuring support during transition, and ensuring that change momentum is maintained.

Process (this phase includes the need for key interpersonal skills such as communication, negotiation, involving and listening):

- Managing up: influencing attitudes and actions of senior managers, negotiating and seeking other forms of commitment and support
- Managing across: securing the cooperation of other departments or external organizations, creating a sense of ownership and using networks
- Managing the team: gaining and keeping motivation and commitment of the change project team members themselves, providing a focus and driving the project, making the most of diversity
- Managing the staff: ensuring the commitment of a wide range of staff upon whom the success of the change ultimately depends, gaining their acceptance and supporting their willingness to be involved.

Control (the purpose of this is to help keep the implementation of change proceeding according to plan with some form of systematic monitoring):

- Keeping track of progress of each phase of the change programme
- Identifying blockages and anticipating delays
- Obtaining acceptable performances from those involved
- Assessing attitudes affecting progress (whether positive or negative)
- Monitoring external changes that have a bearing on change.

Within this there are some specific techniques that could be useful. Some of these are outlined below:

Force field analysis

Force field analysis is a technique developed by Kurt Lewin (Carnall, 1995). It provides a framework based on an idea that any situation can be analysed as a balance between two sets of forces, one opposing the change and one supporting the change. The analysis thus proceeds in four stages:

- Defining the problem in terms of the present situation, with its strengths and weaknesses
- Identifying the forces working for and against the desired changes; the helpers and hinderers, such as people, time and other resources
- Underlining the forces believed to be most important (prioritization),

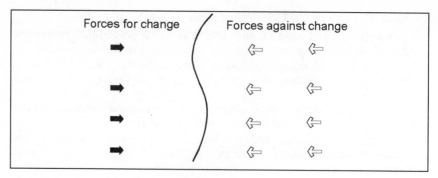

Figure 3.1 Force field analysis.

and listing actions to take, to help change the opposing changes and to strengthen those actions supporting the change
- Agreeing on the actions that appear most likely to help solve the problem, identifying resources and support. This step would be followed by implementation.

A diagram to outline this would look something like Figure 3.1.

Stakeholder analysis

Stakeholder analysis is a technique outlined by Beckhard and Harris (1987). It provides a framework within which all those with a stake (stakeholders) to any change project or task, whether individuals or groups, both internal and external, are identified. Having identified all the stakeholders, their relationship to the change can then be analysed. Four column headings are used as follows:

1. **Impact**. What are the probable consequences? What threats or opportunities arise?
2. **Orientation**. Based on the impact of the change to them (as perceived), are they likely to be for or against the change?
3. **Need**. What is required from this stakeholder for the change to be successful?
4. **Power**. How much power (and what type, e.g. resource power, expert power or information power) does each stakeholder have?

Having highlighted stakeholders' present commitments and the desired commitment required from them for the achievement of the project, this may well provide a picture of where resources and influences are best placed.

Responsibility charting

Responsibility charting (Beckhard and Harris 1987) was developed to assess alternative behaviours for each involved party in a series of actions bringing about change. The chart clarifies the required behaviours to

Table 3.2 The development of clinical effectiveness within self-directed teams

Involved party	Required behaviour
The organization's management team	Approval, informed and support
Team leader	Responsibility and support
Clinical practice facilitator	Support for the team
The team itself	Responsibility and mutual support
Other teams in the trust	Informed
Patients	Informed (where noticeable changes in practice take place)

implement tasks, action or decisions, and helps to reduce ambiguity, clashes, suddenly reduced resources, or interpersonal conflict. The chart is formed by listing those whose roles interrelate, listing actions that affect their relationship. All those who are involved in each action are listed, and then finally the required behaviour for each *actor* is classified on a simple matrix, as:

R = responsibility
A = approval
S = support
I = informed.

This is a useful technique as it also gives a fuller understanding of people's roles involved within the change programme.

An example of how responsibility charting can be started is shown in Table 3.2, using the case study relating to achieving clinical effectiveness via self-directed teams, outlined earlier in this chapter.

PEST and SWOT analyses

PEST analysis provides a simple framework to identify Political, Economic, Sociological and Technological external and environmental factors (Johnson and Scholes, 1993). Under each heading a list is brainstormed and noted. Discussion, analysis of the literature or searches for best practice are used in order to gain a clear picture.

SWOT analysis provides an internal analysis based on Strength, Weakness, Opportunity and Threats. Both PEST and SWOT link together when undertaking an overall analysis.

Ethical issues

In any chapter discussing change it is essential to consider, albeit briefly, the ethical issues involved in undertaking any change.

Twenty-five years ago, business (or management) ethics was not recognized as an academic speciality, but in the 1990s it is. Business ethics emerged because too many businesses lacked a sense of social responsibility, and business people were too frequently prepared to sacrifice ethical concerns to profitability (Shaw, 1996). This may not be quite a parallel to management ethics in healthcare. However, the ethics of managing change are pertinent to all industries.

Wilson and Rosenfeld (1996) cite 'critics of behaviour modification ... there are ethical issues when managers are provided with tools designed to control subordinates. Managers themselves can often feel uncomfortable with the thought of having control over someone else's behaviour'. Managing change is often about changing behaviours. McKendall (1993) states that 'until we look honestly at the natural consequences... we cannot begin to address questions of justice or the questions of organizational versus individual rights'. French and Bell (1990) offer a minimum for ethical standards when involved in organization development or change issues, which can be summarized as:

- Interventions must be selected that have a high probability of being helpful in the particular situation
- The change manager should not use interventions that exceed his or her expertise
- The team or individual should be as informed as is practical about the nature of the process (of change)
- The change manager must not be working with any personal hidden agendas that obtrude into a high quality service for clients
- Commitments to confidentiality must be kept
- Individuals must not be coerced into divulging information about themselves or others
- Unrealistic outcomes must not be promised.

Healthcare managers bear a heavy burden, and ethics sometimes seems a counsel of perfection; it is important to remember that the aim is not to be a saint, but to make better decisions than you would otherwise do if you had not considered the ethical aspects ... (Ovretveit, 1996).

Evaluating change

Finally, and in keeping with the overall purpose of a book on evidence-based healthcare, evaluation is an essential component. New theory can emerge from practice. It is thus important to consider evaluating change practice here.

Organizations must seek to continuously improve. How can improvements be measured? One particular process that can measure improvement is the continuous monitoring and evaluation of change tasks or programmes. Is this the closest link to evidence-based change, the evaluation of effectiveness?

Dictionary definitions (Coulson et al, 1991) tell us that to evaluate means to 'find or state amount or value of ...' and effective is 'having an effect; that is actually brought to bear on an object' or 'the attainment of specific results required by the job through specific actions, consistent with organizational policies'. The problem is that evaluation is to human resource development (or indeed anything) what losing weight is to many people. No one denies its importance, everybody plans to do it, but like losing weight the results are rarely what one had originally hoped for!

Evaluating training and development activities has many models. However, there are not so many for evaluating the effects of change. In 1992, Clement, for example, reported that most published evaluations of organizational development and change efforts were weak, with much reliance on anecdotal reports or other subjective measures, all of which concentrated on output. Recent trends have shown more reliance on the use of harder measures, such as employee productivity, turnover and absenteeism. Paradoxically, change is often poorly evaluated, but is seen to be a good thing!

The evaluation of change should be able to show whether the results of any change programme actually match the programme's intentions. Evaluation will help practitioners to make informed decisions, make the most of scarce resources, and understand whether objectives have been achieved. More specifically, it is important to understand what further areas need work, and understand the costs, and actual impact or consequence of the programme or tasks. The nature of change management requires the use of many models or frameworks. Therefore, change managers or practitioners should be familiar with the use or concept of models and frameworks within their work.

Models for evaluating effectiveness are everything. Using them and being able to equate the outcomes to specific inputs is difficult, particularly while teams or individuals are undergoing a myriad of changes at the same time. However, it is useful to ask three key questions:

1. Did the change programme meet its objectives (validation)?
2. Were these objectives met in the most efficient way (cost-effective analysis)?
3. Was the investment in this intervention worthwhile (cost–benefit analysis)?

Each of these questions can be applied to either individual change, change within a team, or organization-wide change.

More important, however, is the development of criteria by which to measure success. The skill with which one is able to develop criteria will affect the value of the evaluation process itself, thus the key to evaluation is the criterion development phase. Objective setting requires definition, with assurance that perceptions of that definition are the same. These objectives could be short- or long-term, quantitative or qualitative, and may link with other objectives. A common currency should also be used throughout organizations or departments where evaluation is being undertaken, e.g. the profession's or organizational team's definition of effectiveness should be common to all. Many departments painstakingly undertake evaluation only to find that the results are incompatible with one another, and thus some parts of the organization are seen as failures.

The major problem with evaluation is the way words are used within success criteria. Instead of espousing great sentences around becoming more effective, efficient, excellent, etc., more care should be taken to define the x factor within each of these words. One person's definition of improving and another's definition will very likely differ. Careful use of jargon and terminology is paramount. Indeed, the process of exploring these criteria is in itself part of the change process.

Further challenges to bear in mind when evaluating change show that evaluation should start at the beginning of the programme. It forms the basis upon which the programme is developed, and requires full integration. Systematic evaluation gives a continual indication of how things are going. In organizational change there may not be an opportunity to continuously test and retest actions and outcomes. Individuals may move on, as will attitudes and beliefs. Interestingly, many researchers or practitioners do not study the processes of their own interventions, focusing on the outcome only. Process review, reflective practice and evaluation mechanisms make for good change practice. Ultimately, the challenge is to prove what was effective about certain change programme outcomes. This is often difficult because of the complex nature of organizations and the people within them. This may be the difficulty within the search for evidence-based change management.

Summary

There is much written about change management, many tips and hints, frameworks and outlines, tools, techniques and tasks. This chapter has provided a *whistle-stop* tour around some of these. Many writers, as stated previously, advocate change as positive and continuous. However, the problem of evaluation of change is probably the most under-reported issue in British management literature. Perhaps in the journey towards evidence-based healthcare, the full and in-depth evaluation of the process of change within it could provide new ground towards this body of literature?

References

Anderson, N., Hardy, G. and West, M. (1990). Innovative teams at work. *Personnel Management* **22**(9), 48, 50–1.

Beckhard, R. and Harris, R. T. (1987). *Organisational Transitions: Managing Complex Change*. Addison-Wesley.

Belbin, M. (1981). *Management Teams: Why They Succeed or Fail*. Heinemann.

Buchanan, D. A. and Boddy, D. (1992). *The Expertise of the Change Agent: Public Performance and Backstage Activity*. Prentice-Hall.

Bulletpoint (1994). *Change Management Issue 14*. Bulletpoint.

Burnes, B. (1992). *Managing Change*. Pitman.

Carnall, C. (1995). *Managing Change in Organizations*. Prentice-Hall.

Clement, R. W. (1992). The changing face of organisation development: views of a manager turned academic. *Business Horizons*, **May–June**, 6–12.

Coulson, J., Carr, C., Hutchinson, L., et al. (1991). *Oxford Illustrated Dictionary*. Book Club Associates.

Covey, S. (1989). *Seven Habits of Highly Effective People*. Simon & Schuster.

Department of Health. (1997). *The New NHS: Modern, Dependable*. Stationery Office.

French, W. and Bell, J. R. (1990). *Organisation Development: Behavioural Science Interventions for Organisation Improvement*. Prentice-Hall.

Johnson, G. and Scholes, K. (1993). *Exploring Corporate Strategy*. Prentice-Hall.

Lewin, K. (1958). Group decision and social change. In *Readings in Social Psychology* (E. Maccoby, T. Newcomb and E. Hartley, eds). Holt Rhinehart & Winston.

Lindenfield, G. (1992). *The Positive Women*. Harper Collins.

Margerison, C. and McCann, D. (1990). *Team Management: Practical New Approaches*. Mercury Books.

Marshall, J. (1995). *Women Managers Moving On*. Routledge.

McKendall, M. (1993). The tyranny of change: organizational development revisited. *Journal of Business Ethics*, **12**, 93–104.

Ovretveit, J. (1996). Ethics: a counsel of perfection. *IHSM Network*, **3**(13), 4–50.

Rogers, C. R. (1967). *On Becoming a Person*. Constable.

Salaman, G. C. (1992). *Human Resource Strategies*. Sage.

Shaw, W. H. (1996). Business ethics today: a survey. *Journal of Business Ethics*, **15**, 489–500.

Vann Gennep, A. (1960). *The Rites of Passage*. Routledge & Kegan Paul.

Wilson, D. and Rosenfeld, R. H. (1996). *Managing Organisations*. Routledge.

4

Getting research into practice: changing behaviour

Tracy Bury

Introduction

This book promotes an evidence-based approach to healthcare, encouraging practitioners, managers, purchasers and policy-makers to base what they do on research evidence, where it exists. The previous chapter has discussed various approaches to the management of change. This chapter sets out specific strategies for getting research into practice which have been subject to evaluation. Research sets out to generate theories and to develop knowledge and understanding. It also aims to make a difference, so it is important that the end point for research is not simply publication, but improvements in patient care and health services.

> There are no 'magic bullets' for improving the quality of health care. There are, however, a wide range of interventions available that, if used appropriately, could lead to substantial improvements in clinical care derived from the best available evidence. (Oxman et al, 1995)

The strategies for implementing the findings of good-quality research constitute an area of investigation in their own right. In recognition of this, there has been a dedicated programme of research funded by the NHS Research and Development (R&D) Programme (Department of Health, 1995). Also, as part of the Cochrane Collaboration (described in Chapter 6), there is a review group looking at Effective Practice and Organisation of Care (EPOC) and strategies for changing the behaviour of all healthcare professionals (Freemantle et al, 1995).

This chapter outlines the processes of diffusion, dissemination and implementation. An overview of the systematic reviews evaluating strategies for changing practitioner behaviour to implement research findings is then presented. Advice is given on how this information can inform the facilitation of change in relation to specific interventions. This provides you with some principles and options for changing practitioner behaviour at a local level. This is complementary to the area of organizational change presented in the previous chapter, the use of clinical guidelines covered in Chapter 8 and clinical audit described in Chapter 9.

Diffusion, dissemination and implementation

Before research is implemented in practice it usually goes through processes of diffusion and dissemination. Publishing information alone, such as a journal publication or a flyer in a professional magazine, is rarely sufficient to change practice. This needs to be complemented with strategies specifically targeted at implementation. These strategies need to be sustainable over time and flexible enough to accommodate changes in the evidence.

Diffusion

Diffusion is a passive process which is largely uncontrolled and unplanned (Lomas, 1993). Researchers strive to gain publication of their work in peer-reviewed scientific journals. They are selective in where they choose to publish. This tends to be associated with the academic credibility of the journal and the audience they are trying to influence. Once published, the research **may** be incorporated into continuing education and undergraduate courses, other information formats and changes in practice. This is more likely to happen when individuals are active in seeking out information (Lomas, 1993).

The work of Turner and Whitfield (1996, 1997) suggests that this active seeking out of information does not reflect the behaviour of physiotherapists. In a survey of journal readership in the UK, they found that the *Physiotherapy* journal, which is mailed to all subscribing members of the Chartered Society of Physiotherapy (CSP), was read on average five to six times over a six-month period. Readership of other journals was limited to two or fewer over the same period of time (Turner and Whitfield, 1996). However, reading was not defined and might have been interpreted by respondents as anything from scanning the contents list to a more in-depth consideration of an article. The authors pointed out the concern that the primary source of research literature read was a generalist journal. In a later study, they found that over 90 per cent of the interventions used by physiotherapists, surveyed in the UK and Australia, reflected what was taught in undergraduate education. Research literature was ranked the lowest (less than 30 per cent of respondents) as a basis for choosing an intervention approach (Turner and Whitfield, 1997). From this research, the role of educationalists, in keeping abreast of the research literature and facilitating the transfer of research to practice, was highlighted. There is nothing to suggest that their findings do not apply to other therapists. Also, it should not be assumed that when practitioners read the research literature they are able to select and critically appraise the evidence, and use it appropriately to guide their clinical decisions.

Diffusion alone will only be effective if:

- Individuals are already actively seeking out information
- Individuals are highly motivated
- The rewards from finding the evidence are high
- There is a relatively small pool of information to minimize search costs (Lomas, 1993).

Dissemination

The overall aims of a **dissemination** strategy are to make research information more easily accessible and to target it more appropriately. In doing so, greater efforts are made to raise awareness and prepare individuals for change. Researchers are becoming more active participants in this process, with conference presentations and the outputs of research being made available via a variety of media. However, it should not be assumed that dissemination alone is sufficient to change practice (Haines and Jones, 1994).

Efforts have been made to present relevant, high-quality information in a concise format for research users, sifting out irrelevant and poor-quality material. Systematic reviews, such as those included in the Cochrane Library, mentioned in Chapter 6, and clinical guidelines, described in Chapter 8, are good examples of how the research evidence can be synthesized. Dissemination strategies are often on a national scale, for example the publication of an *Effective Health Care Bulletin* (see Chapter 6).

Implementation

Having disseminated the research information into the public domain, further work is required to **implement** the necessary changes in practice.

> There are unacceptable delays in the implementation of many findings of research. This results in suboptimal care for patients. (Haines and Jones, 1994)

Healthcare professionals work in a world with competing demands and different agendas. Consideration needs to be given to how the research evidence can be promoted to them and mechanisms established to assist with the change process. It will need to be embedded into channels that will influence the individuals concerned. Information to facilitate implementation is best presented with details of the implications of the research for a defined audience clearly highlighted (Lomas, 1993). Implementation strategies are generally local, because of the need to address issues that are dependent on local circumstances. A good example of this is the local adaptation of national clinical guidelines described in Chapter 8.

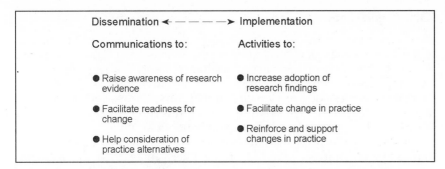

Figure 4.1 Continuum of change. (Reproduced from NHS Centre for Reviews and Dissemination (1996) CRD Report 4, with permission.)

Bringing dissemination and implementation together

Dissemination and implementation approaches can be seen as a continuum (NHS Centre for Reviews and Dissemination, 1996) as shown in Figure 4.1. It is difficult to see how implementation can be achieved without awareness having been raised through dissemination. These approaches are reflected in the activities discussed in the next section.

Interventions to facilitate change

What interventions have been used to change the behaviour of healthcare professionals? Research to date has focused on strategies to implement research and change behaviour for general patient management, preventative services, drug prescribing, conditions such as hypertension and diabetes mellitus, diagnostic services and hospital utilization (Oxman et al, 1995). Most of this has focused on changing the behaviour of doctors and, to a lesser extent, nurses. While therapists have not been involved in these investigations, it should still be possible to apply the lessons learnt. How these might apply to managers, purchasers or policy-makers is less clear. The following interventions have been evaluated:

- Clinical guidelines
- Educational approaches
- Audit and feedback
- Outreach visits
- Conferences
- Local opinion leaders
- Patient-mediated interventions
- Reminder or computerized decision support systems
- Local consensus processes
- Marketing
- Multifaceted interventions.

Each of these will be examined in more detail.

Clinical guidelines

Few can have failed to notice the increasing emphasis on clinical guidelines. The use of clinical guidelines is discussed in detail in Chapter 8. The publication of a clinical guideline is rarely sufficient to change practice. Clinical guidelines often have the advantage of involving a number of professions and cover different care settings, such as primary and secondary care. This may be more influential in bringing about change that requires collective action (Haines et al, 1996).

Reviews of the implementation of clinical guidelines provide some indication of strategies that are more likely to lead to the intended changes in practice (Grimshaw and Russell, 1993; Nuffield Institute for Health, 1994). These are summarized in Table 4.1. It is unfortunate that the conclusions of these reviews were limited due to the nature and quality of the original studies evaluated. However, strategies closely associated with practice and the end-user are more likely to be effective.

Table 4.1 Strategies to implement clinical guidelines

Unsuccessful	Successful

Dissemination strategies alone:
    Publication in a professional journal
	Active implementation strategies:
	    Educational outreach visits
	    Use of local opinion leaders
	    Patient-mediated interventions
	    Patient-specific reminders in
	    consultations

Educational approaches

Reviews by Davis et al (1992, 1995) have examined a wide range of **educational approaches**. They used a broad definition of educational approaches as any attempt to persuade practitioners to modify their practice performance by communicating clinical information. Table 4.2 provides an indication of the success of various interventions.

When two of the effective strategies were combined, positive changes resulted. However, combining less effective strategies resulted in mixed results. A major weakness included in many of the original studies was the omission of change in patient outcomes, the primary outcome being change in practitioner behaviour.

The use of **educational material** to improve the behaviour of healthcare professionals and patient outcomes has been examined by Freemantle et al (1998). They found that their use alone appeared to be limited and that the value of additional strategies remained unclear. The use of **outreach visits** and **opinion leaders**, in conjunction with **printed materials**, seemed promising, but the authors were unable to make firm conclusions because of the limited number of studies and the relatively poor quality.

Table 4.2 Educational approaches to changing clinician behaviour

Least success	⟶	Most success
Continuing education activities, e.g. conferences	Audit and feedback Educational materials	Reminders Patient-mediated interventions Outreach visits Use of opinion leaders Multifaceted interventions

In a systematic review investigating the effect of training health professionals to provide smoking cessation interventions, Silagy and colleagues (1995) found that those professionals who had received specific training were more likely to perform tasks of smoking cessation than untrained controls. There was an increase in the number of patients receiving counselling and setting quit dates, and more were given self-help materials and follow-up appointments. The effectiveness of this approach was improved if it was combined with **prompts** and **reminders**. Overall they concluded that training health professionals to provide smoking cessation interventions had a measurable impact on professional performance, but only a modest effect on patient outcome. They suggest that further studies are required to investigate the effectiveness of training different health professionals, such as physiotherapists, who are well placed to facilitate smoking cessation. This research would need to take account of the working patterns and behaviours of different professions and the different environments within which the smoking cessation strategies could be used. Physiotherapists are already involved in advising about lifestyle changes as part of interventions, and perhaps the smoking cessation advice would be incorporated into an overall healthy lifestyle package, providing a holistic approach.

Strategies for implementing changes in **primary care** have been reviewed by Wensing and Grol (1994). They found that the use of educational materials did not result in improvements in care. However, **individual instruction** did appear to be effective. Group education combined with different strategies, such as **feedback** and the provision of materials (practice support) was also shown to be effective. The authors felt that the use of educational materials and group education, directed at skills competency, may have achieved only modest effects because they only focused on barriers to change concerning skills.

Audit and feedback

Oxman and colleagues (1995) used a broad definition of **audit and feedback** which encompasses any summary of clinical performance of healthcare provided over a specified period of time, with or without recommendations for clinical action. This should not be confused with clinical audit as detailed in Chapter 9. Information may have been collected via a variety of tools, such as patient records or observation. A

Table 4.3 Effectiveness of audit and feedback approaches

Less effective	*More effective*
Passive	Active
Unsolicited provision of information	Clinicians engaged in the process
No stated action plan	The need to review practice already agreed by decision-makers
	Information provided close to the time of decision-making
	Person in authority provides individual feedback

number of reviews have assessed the effectiveness of audit and feedback (Lomas et al, 1991; Mugford et al, 1991; Thomson et al, 1998b, 1998c). The results from these are summarized in Table 4.3.

Audit and feedback do improve the performance of healthcare professionals, but only to a small or moderate extent (Thomson et al, 1998a). Lessons still need to be learnt about how varying the different characteristics of audit and feedback might impact on their success (Thomson et al, 1998b).

Outreach visits

The term **outreach visits** is used to describe the use of a trained person who meets with practitioners in their practice setting. It has primarily been used to improve the prescribing practice of physicians. The trained individual provides information to meet defined objectives and may provide feedback on the provider's performance (Oxman et al, 1995).

While the term outreach visits may not be familiar to therapists, a comparison can be made with commercial representatives from equipment companies. New equipment and products appear at regular intervals. These representatives know their product and should also be informed about developmental work and any research relating to it. They may leave equipment on trial in departments and provide feedback to users. However, there are a number of concerns:

- The products have not necessarily been developed through stringent research processes
- The training and level of knowledge of the representative may be limited
- The motive could be more commercially driven than a desire to change practice and improve patient outcomes based on research evidence.

Also, unsystematic trial periods in departments are not a suitable way of demonstrating the effectiveness of equipment.

In a recent review of 18 trials of outreach visits, positive effects on practice were observed in all trials (Thomson et al, 1998c). The visits consisted of several components including **written materials** and

conferences. Some were supplemented by audit and feedback. The authors were not able to identify the key characteristics of outreach visits important for success. The use of such visits appeared to be most successful when combined with **social marketing** (described later in this section) and aimed at drug prescribing behaviour.

Interviews to assess baseline knowledge, motivation and barriers to change may be a key component to success. The use of such visits is costly and further research is required to identify which components contribute to their effectiveness (Thomson et al, 1998c).

Conferences

The use of **conferences** has been reviewed by Oxman and colleagues (1995). They included many of the classical continuing education approaches:

- Conferences
- Workshops
- Lectures.

Not surprisingly, considering that dissemination-only approaches do not make explicit efforts to determine practice needs or facilitate practice change, they found that performance and healthcare outcomes failed to improve. However, where **workshops** were part of a more comprehensive package, including **patient education** and **practice-reinforcing** strategies, changes in practice did result.

It is interesting to consider this in light of current continuing education activities, which are primarily chosen by practitioners themselves, often to meet the requirements of posts or the expectations of managers and peers. This often requires attendance at named courses so that they can be included on a curriculum vitae. Approaches to professional development need to consider carefully how competency to practice can be assured, given the lack of evidence to support the use of conferences and lectures in changing practitioner behaviour. The distinction should be drawn between attendance and the resulting quality of learning and impact on behaviour, skills and practice.

Local opinion leaders

The use of local **opinion leaders** is probably familiar to therapists. It refers to the use of practitioners identified by their colleagues as 'educationally influential' (Oxman et al, 1995). A review by Thomson and colleagues (1998d) of six trials, examined the influence of local opinion leaders in a number of patient problems, including osteoarthritis, rheumatoid arthritis, chronic lung disease and vaginal birth after previous caesarian section. They found mixed results, with five of the trials showing an improvement in healthcare professional practice. Only one of the three trials, which evaluated the impact on patient outcome, resulted in a practical improvement. While the authors were unable to conclude what local opinion leaders actually do, the following might influence their success:

- Their ability to influence the attitudes and behaviour of others
- Their level of knowledge and competence concerning the intervention
- Their credibility and status among colleagues
- Their knowledge of local circumstances and barriers.

They also suggested that an opinion leader in one environment may not be influential in another.

The use of local opinion leaders has been compared with audit and feedback in getting obstetricians to follow clinical guidelines for the management of women who have had a previous caesarian section. The obstetricians were able to identify the local opinion leaders used in the educational approach. In this instance, local opinion leaders were found to be more successful in reducing caesarian rates than mailed clinical guidelines or audit and feedback (Lomas et al, 1991).

Patient-mediated interventions

In this approach the patient becomes the **change agent**. Patients are presented with information about the effectiveness of interventions in order to influence the behaviour of the health professionals, thereby improving their own health outcomes. Much of the work is derived from the fields of smoking cessation and diabetes mellitus (Oxman et al, 1995). This strategy appears to be more successful when used as part of a multifaceted intervention.

A systematic review is underway to examine the impact of **mass media campaigns** on health services utilization and healthcare outcomes (Grilli et al, 1998). The results of this review are expected towards the end of 1998. Mass media includes all channels of communication aimed at reaching a large number of people: radio, television, newspapers, magazines, leaflets, poster pamphlets, etc. The use of the media is an established health promotion strategy. Campaigns linked to smoking, drinking and diet are familiar to all. Increasingly, research articles on health issues, published in scientific journals, are used by the media to inform the public. In doing so, reports may (Grilli et al, 1998):

- Increase or diminish the willingness of individuals to present for care
- Raise expectations (appropriately or otherwise)
- Dash hopes
- Provoke alarm.

Caution should be used in evaluating information presented in the media, as those preparing news items may not be skilled in critical appraisal, and therefore may selectively convey certain healthcare messages. Researchers and those responsible for implementing research findings would do well to collaborate actively with the media to try to ensure that messages are conveyed accurately and responsibly.

Reminders and computerized decision support systems

Manual or **computerized prompts** have been used to remind providers to perform certain actions (Oxman et al, 1995). A systematic review by Johnston and colleagues (1994) showed that computerized decision support systems can improve practitioner performance, but further conclusions were limited due to a lack of information on patient outcomes in the original research. They defined a **clinical decision support system** (CDSS) as computer software using a knowledge base designed for use by a practitioner involved in patient care, as a direct aid to clinical decision-making. The studies included involved drug doses, aids to diagnosis, and preventative or active medical care. Studies using CDSS showed that they were more effective for preventative or active medical care than as an aid to diagnosis.

The use of prompt systems has yet to be investigated among therapists. With the current state of information technology among these professions, it is likely that prompt systems would need to be in manual formats primarily, such as reminders attached to notes, until information technology improves.

Local consensus processes

A **local consensus process** involves providers meeting to agree a clinical problem, the strategy for managing it and the necessary action (Oxman et al, 1995). It is an approach that may sound familiar to therapists. There has been little evaluation work in this area, and the review by Oxman and colleagues (1995) was unable to draw any firm conclusions.

One of the problems of this approach is the likelihood of bias being introduced. From the discussion in Chapter 1, on types and strengths of evidence, you will recall that opinion is the least reliable form of evidence. Within the hierarchy presented, opinion referred to that of respected authorities, based on clinical evidence, descriptive studies or reports of expert committees (Moore et al, 1995). This would not necessarily be reflected in the process of establishing opinion at a local level. It would depend on what efforts were made to track down the available evidence. In the absence of any research evidence, opinion based on clinical experience may be the best available information. An important first step, irrespective of the strategy then used to develop consensus, is to gain agreement between local practitioners that the problem is an important one.

Marketing

Marketing involves identifying barriers to change and then developing an intervention to facilitate change. This approach has been closely linked to continuing education strategies and the use of outreach visits (Davis et al, 1995; Oxman et al, 1995; Thomson et al, 1998c). **Social marketing** has been categorized by Soumerai and Avorn (1990) as an eight step process:

1. Interviews to assess baseline knowledge, motivation for current practice and barriers to change
2. Developing programmes for specific practitioner targets and their opinion leaders
3. Developing clear educational and behavioural objectives
4. Establishing credibility of the information by presenting both sides of issues
5. Encouraging practitioner participation in educational interactions
6. Using concise educational materials
7. Repeating key messages
8. Providing positive reinforcement through subsequent visits.

In Davis and colleagues' (1995) review of continuing medical education strategies, they attempted to determine the extent to which interventions were planned as a result of an analysis of practice identifying barriers to change. They concluded that 'when barriers to change were addressed or gaps were demonstrated and resources deployed to help the learner, change appeared to occur relatively frequently'. This would appear to support the effectiveness of marketing interventions in conjunction with other approaches.

Multifaceted interventions

This refers to a combination of approaches using two or more of the strategies already described (Oxman et al, 1995). Many of the interventions have been used in a wide range of combinations. It is because of the possible combinations that it is difficult to interpret studies of this nature as there is very little overlap or consistent approach. However, it would appear that multifaceted interventions tend to be more successful than single approaches, although combining less effective single strategies does not appear to improve their effectiveness.

In Wensing and Grol's (1994) review of implementation strategies in primary care, the most effective approaches were individual instruction combined with another approach and the use of peer review and feedback.

Putting it into practice to facilitate change

Initiating change

As has already been emphasized, the success of change strategies is likely to be closely linked to identifying barriers to change and the selection of the most appropriate approach(es). Barriers to change will vary from one situation to another. The previous chapter has covered this in detail. Personal, environmental and behavioural factors, as well as the nature of the intervention being introduced, will all influence the change process (Bandura, 1977, 1986; Fox et al, 1989).

As Oxman and colleagues (1995) said, '... there is a need in the area of health professional performance to include appropriate diagnostic strategies (to determine the reasons for suboptimal performance and to identify barriers to change) and to select carefully the interventions most likely to be effective in light of the diagnosed problem'.

What is likely to trigger a change leading to the adoption of research evidence in practice?

- A question arising from practice/services
- Someone is aware of the need to change practice
- Variations in practice
- Awareness of a new intervention.

The awareness, attitudes, beliefs, values and knowledge of practitioners may be altered by information that enters their environment, motivating them to initiate change (Green et al, 1980; Green and Eriksen, 1988). Prompts will alert practitioners to a need to consider change and include active dissemination approaches. An *Effective Health Care Bulletin*, clinical guideline or research article are all possible prompts.

Understanding how people change

If only people were rational! Why, when presented with clear unambiguous information that sets out the facts, does rational action not always follow? You only have to look at the areas of addiction, such as smoking and alcohol, or lifestyle changes such as exercise and diet, to know that change does not simply follow information, even if the implications of action or inaction are clear. How and why individuals change is complex. In attempting to change health professional behaviour, there is much that can be learnt from the fields of psychology and health promotion.

Therapists may be familiar with the **readiness for change** model of Prochaska and DiClemente (1986). It was primarily developed for addictive behaviours. It is based on the theory that people move through an orderly sequence of change, at different paces. Some may get stuck at certain points or even regress. The stages are:

1. **Precontemplation**: those who have no intention to change their behaviour. Individuals do not seek out information or re-evaluate their personal behaviours. They are also less receptive to others who may wish to discuss the problem.
2. **Contemplation**: thinking about change. Re-evaluating personal circumstances, attitudes and beliefs are important steps for contemplators. They are more likely to retrieve information and pursue educational activities.
3. **Action**: change behaviour. For success it is vital that individuals act from a belief that they have the autonomy to change their behaviour,

as opposed to an external force determining the change. It is also necessary that they have the appropriate skills required for the new behaviour.

4. **Maintenance**: successfully sustain behaviour change. This builds on the previous stages.

Both action and maintenance will benefit from the support of others and appropriate reinforcement.

This model provides an insight into how people change their behaviour and the requirements to move from one stage to the next. However, different people respond to the introduction of new ideas in different ways. Rogers (1983) defined five categories of people:

1. **Innovators**: a small group who may be distrusted by others.
2. **Early adopters**: respected, approachable opinion leaders.
3. **Early majority**: those who hold traditional values and are capable of change. They often provide the peer pressure to help the late majority change.
4. **Late majority**: sceptics reluctant to change.
5. **Laggards**: the diehards!

Do you identify with one of these categories, or recognize colleagues in the descriptions? Think how this might alter the dynamics of the change process.

Opinion leaders have already been acknowledged as being influential in implementing evidence in practice. The rate of uptake of an intervention will be influenced by the effect that they have on their colleagues (Haines and Jones, 1994). They are the early adopters identified by Rogers.

During the contemplation stage, while considering and thinking about action, important factors may influence the individual:

- The belief that by changing their behaviour they can produce the desired effect, called **outcome efficacy expectations**
- The belief that they have the skills and are competent to perform the behaviour, referred to as **self-efficacy expectations** (Bandura, 1977, 1986).

Individuals may also be influenced by the decisions and beliefs of colleagues, the early adopters, when evaluating new information and its implication for behaviour (Mittman et al, 1992). This recognizes that individuals do not change in isolation, but are part of a social grouping.

How an individual feels about a change will influence his or her move to the action phase. When social pressure to change behaviour is present, such as peer pressure from respected colleagues, change is more likely, especially when combined with intention to change (Ajzen and Fishbein, 1980), although it is important that individuals perceive that they have control over their actions as well. Personal motivation for change is better than professional motivation, which in turn is better than external and social motivators as the forces driving change (Fox et al, 1989).

Selecting the intervention to implement

It is not possible to introduce more than one significant change at any one time. When trying to implement research evidence, it is important to start by choosing an intervention that you are more likely to be successful at introducing. Certain features of an intervention will influence its uptake (Rogers, 1983):

- Its **relative advantage**, for the practitioner and patient care. The new intervention will be compared with an existing one to weigh up the likely improvement
- The new intervention's **compatibility** with personal values and past experience, reflecting established practice
- How **complex** the intervention is to understand and introduce
- The opportunity to introduce the intervention for a **trial** period and to stop using it if it is found to be inappropriate, thereby providing a test period without committing resources indefinitely
- The easier it is to **observe** the anticipated results, the more likely it is that the intervention will be adopted.

Before proceeding, it is useful to use this list as a way of clearly identifying the characteristics of the intervention. It needs to be feasible to introduce and adaptable to local circumstances, without changing it beyond recognition or tampering with the evidence. No matter what the impetus for change, or source of evidence, it is important to be clear that this is the right intervention to be introducing at this time. Chapter 9 also provides some guidance on prioritizing topics for implementation, such as the use of quality impact analysis.

Designing the implementation programme

The previous chapter should have prepared you to deal with change, keeping a broad perspective of the many interdependent factors. Within this context, the specific strategies to implement research evidence into practice can be incorporated.

Enabling factors usually focus on overcoming barriers to change that result from forces within the local community. Examples of barriers might be educational, administrative, economic, community-based, patient-based, or personal. Approaches therefore need to be local and personalized, building on established predisposing factors (Green et al, 1980; Green and Eriksen, 1988). Table 4.4 provides some examples of the strategies that are likely to be more successful in addressing specific barriers identified.

It is likely that more than one barrier will be present when an intervention is being implemented; this supports the need for multi-faceted approaches. Consideration also needs to be given to which staff should be involved. This may need to be staged, working with the early adopters and early majority first. Do not start by putting a lot of time and effort into working with the laggards and those at the precontemplation stage. You need to work with those from whom you can expect change,

Table 4.4 Matching strategies to barriers

Barrier	Strategy
Lack of knowledge/skills	Educational training and peer support
Evidence exists, but is not available when required	Reminders
Lack of respect for evidence	Influential opinion leader to endorse change
Lack of awareness of evidence	Dissemination strategies including educational material, group discussions
Individuals do not agree that their performance needs to change (below par)	Counselling sessions, peer support
Problems maintaining change	Audit and feedback

thereby demonstrating beneficial outcomes as a mechanism of persuasion and marketing the intervention to others.

Resources required for the specific implementation strategy need to have been fully considered, along with the resource implications of providing the new intervention, before embarking on a change programme.

Principles for successful implementation

Common features for successful change emerge from the literature:

- Local **opinion leaders** are influential and need to be identified by the practitioners concerned with the change
- There needs to be **flexibility** in how the innovation is introduced to allow for adaptation to local conditions
- The intervention needs to be **marketed** to practitioners in a way that accounts for the realities of practice, allows **needs** to be assessed and **barriers** identified
- Individuals need to be **ready to change** and take some responsibility for their actions
- They need to have the **skills** to affect the change and be competent in their use, believing that they can bring about the anticipated outcome
- Implementation is facilitated by all members of the **social grouping**, whether uniprofessional or multiprofessional, working together
- Change is more likely when the new intervention does not diverge too much from established practice.

Maintaining change

There can be a number of reasons why an intervention, once implemented, does not become established practice:

- Lack of resources
- Practitioners lapsing back into previous habits
- Practitioners are not satisfied with the results arising from the new intervention and revert to that which they consider improves outcomes
- The practitioners' beliefs are driving practice.

Audit and feedback are important in evaluating that the change has resulted in the anticipated improvements in practice. Useful mechanisms for providing feedback, both negative and positive, act as reinforcement for the change, where this is appropriate.

Rogers (1983) described the successful maintenance of change as **confirmation**. The new intervention is accepted as established practice.

Reinforcing factors reward and maintain changes (Green et al, 1980; Green and Eriksen, 1988). Audit and feedback, reminder systems, opinion leaders and media campaigns are all examples of reinforcing strategies.

Summary

This chapter has highlighted the variety of strategies that exist to facilitate the implementation of research in practice. While all have their merits, the evidence to support their effectiveness is stronger for some approaches than for others. Those where there is stronger evidence of effectiveness are educational outreach visits and multifaceted interventions. Audit and feedback and the use of local opinion leaders have resulted in mixed effects. The least effective strategies appear to be didactic educational sessions and the distribution of printed materials alone. This may be linked to the fact that experiential, or informal, learning is more closely associated with personal motivators, whereas formal, more didactic, learning is linked to professional motivators and compliance with external influences (Fox et al, 1989).

While dissemination strategies alone are rarely enough to change practice, it is important to recognize that they are invariably the initial step in bringing new interventions to the attention of some health professionals. The research needs to have been synthesized by a respectable body and disseminated in an accessible format which highlights the benefit of change in comparison to current practice. This is an important message for those responsible for disseminating research information.

Those responsible for change need to appreciate the important relationship between barriers to change and effective implementation strategies. This omission may explain the relative ineffectiveness of some of the strategies discussed earlier. To be successful, implementation strategies need to address the barriers that exist, and they need to be used in a multifaceted approach determined by these barriers.

Understanding how individuals change in response to healthcare information has been investigated primarily in relation to patients and the general public, but provides an insight into how health professionals are likely to change practice. Considerable research exists investigating the effectiveness of change strategies, but further work is required to establish key features of successful interventions and combinations. Work to date has not included the therapy professions as the focus of change. While there is nothing to suggest that lessons from the medical field can not be applied to therapists, their structure and organizational environment differ, which highlights a need for specific research in this area.

Acknowledgements

Jacqueline Droogan and Ian Watt provided helpful comments on an early draft of this chapter.

References

Ajzen, I. and Fishbein, M. (1980). *Understanding Attitudes and Predicting Social Behaviour.* Prentice-Hall.

Bandura, A. (1977). *Social Learning Theory.* Prentice-Hall.

Bandura, A. (1986). *Social Foundations of Thought and Action: A Social Cognitive Theory.* Prentice-Hall.

Davis, D. A., Thomson, M. A., Oxman, A. D., et al. (1992). Evidence for the effectiveness of CME: a review of 50 randomized controlled trials. *JAMA*, **268**(9), 1111–7.

Davis, D. A., Thomson, M. A., Oxman, A. D. and Haynes, R. B. (1995). Changing physician performance: a systematic review of the effect of continuing medical education strategies. *JAMA*, **274**(9), 700–5.

Department of Health (1995). *Methods to Promote the Implementation of Research Findings in the NHS – Priorities for Evaluation.* Department of Health.

Fox, R., Mazmanian, P. and Putnam, R.W. (1989). *Changing and Learning in the Lives of Physicians.* Praeger.

Freemantle, N., Grilli, R., Grimshaw, J., et al. (1995). Implementing findings of medical research: the Cochrane Collaboration on Effective Professional Practice. *Qual Health Care,* **5**, 45–7.

Freemantle, N., Harvey, E. L., Wolf, F., et al. (1998). Printed educational materials to improve the behaviour of health care professionals and patient outcomes. In *Cochrane Collaboration on Effective Professional Practice Module of the Cochrane Database of Systematic Reviews* [updated 01 December 1997] (L. Bero, R. Grilli, J. Grimshaw, and A. Oxman, eds). Available in The Cochrane Library [database on disk and CDROM]. The Cochrane Collaboration, issue 1. Oxford: Update Software, 1998 [updated quarterly].

Green, L., Kreuter, M., Deeds, S., et al. (1980). *Health Education Planning: A Diagnostic Approach.* Mayfield Press.

Green, L. W. and Eriksen, M. P. (1988). Behavioural determinants of preventative practices by physicians. *Am J Prev Med*, **4**(suppl), 101–7.

Grilli, R., Minozzi, S., Freemantle, N., et al. (1998). The impact of mass media campaigns on health services utilisation and health outcomes [protocol]. In *Cochrane Collaboration on Effective Professional Practice Module of the Cochrane Database of Systematic Reviews* [updated 01 December 1997] (L. Bero, R. Grilli, J. Grimshaw, and A. Oxman, eds). Available in the Cochrane Library [database on disk and CDROM]. The Cochrane Collaboration, issue 1. Oxford: Update Software, 1998 [updated quarterly].

Grimshaw, J. M. and Russell, I. T. (1993). Achieving health gain through clinical guidelines. II: ensuring that guidelines change medical practice. *Qual Health Care*, **3**, 45–52.

Haines, A., Freemantle, N., Watt, I., et al. (1996). Increasing the effectiveness of clinical intervention. In *Effective Clinical Practice*. (A. Miles and M. Lugon, eds) pp. 124–43, Blackwell Science.

Haines, A. and Jones, R. (1994). Implementing findings of research. *BMJ*, **308**, 1488–92.

Johnston, M. E., Langton, K. B., Haynes, R. B., et al. (1994). Effects of computer-based clinical decision-support systems on clinician performance and patient outcome. A critical appraisal of research. *Ann Intern Med*, **120**(2), 135–42.

Lomas, J. (1993). Diffusion, dissemination and implementation: who should do what? In *Doing More Good than Harm: the Evaluation of Health Care Interventions*. (K. Warren and F. Mosteller, eds). *N Y Acad Sci*, **703**, 226–35.

Lomas, J., Enkin, M., Anderson, G. M., et al. (1991). Opinion leaders vs audit and feedback to implement practice guidelines. Delivery after previous cesarean section. *JAMA*, **265**(17), 2202–7.

Mittman, B., Tonesk, X. and Jacobson, P. (1992). Implementing clinical practice guidelines: social influence strategies and practitioner behaviour change. *Qual Rev Bull*, **18**, 413–22.

Moore, A., McQuay, H. and Gray, J. A. M. (eds) (1995). Evidence-based everything. *Bandolier*, **1**(12), 1.

Mugford, M., Banfield, P. and O'Hanlon, M. (1991). Effects of feedback of information on clinical practice: a review. *BMJ*, **303**, 398–402.

NHS Centre for Reviews and Dissemination (1996). *Undertaking Systematic Reviews of Research in Effectiveness. CRD Guidelines For Those Carrying Out or Commissioning Reviews*. CRD Report 4. University of York.

Nuffield Institute for Health (1994). *Effective Health Care. Implementing Clinical Guidelines*. Bulletin no. 8. University of Leeds.

Oxman, A., Thomson, M. A., Davis, D. A. and Haynes, R. B. (1995). No magic bullets: a systematic review of 102 trials of interventions to improve professional practice. *Can Med Assoc J*, **153**(10), 1423–31.

Prochaska, J. and DiClemente, C. (1986). Towards a comprehensive model of change. In *Treating Addictive Behaviour: Processes of Change*. (W. Miller and N. Heather, eds). pp. 33–62, Plenum Press.

Rogers, E. M. (1983). *Diffusion of Innovations*. Free Press.

Silagy, C., Lancaster, T., Gray, S., et al. (1995). The effectiveness of training health professionals to provide smoking cessation interventions: systematic review of randomised controlled trials. *Qual Health Care*, **3**, 193–8.

Soumerai, S. B. and Avorn, J. (1990). Principles of educational outreach ('academic detailing') to improve clinical decision making. *JAMA*, **263**(4), 549–56.

Thomson, M. A., Oxman, A. D., Davis, D. A., et al. (1998a). Audit and feedback to improve health professional practice and health care outcomes (part I). In *Cochrane Collaboration on Effective Professional Practice Module of the Cochrane Database of Systematic Reviews* [updated 01 December 1997] (L. Bero, R. Grilli, J. Grimshaw and A. Oxman, eds). Available in The Cochrane Library [database on disk and CDROM]. The Cochrane Collaboration, issue 1. Oxford: Update Software, 1998 [updated quarterly].

Thomson, M. A., Oxman, A. D., Davis, D. A., et al. (1998b). Audit and feedback to improve health professional practice and health care outcomes (part II). In *Cochrane Collaboration* on *Effective Professional Practice Module of the Cochrane Database of Systematic Reviews* [updated 01 December 1997] (L. Bero, R. Grilli, J. Grimshaw and A. Oxman, eds). Available in The Cochrane Library [database on disk and CDROM]. The Cochrane Collaboration, issue 1. Oxford: Update Software, 1998 [updated quarterly].

Thomson, M. A., Oxman, A. D., Davis, D., et al. (1998c). Outreach visits to improve health care professional practice and health care outcomes. In *Cochrane Collaboration on Effective Professional Practice Module of the Cochrane Database of Systematic Reviews* [updated 01 December 1997] (L. Bero, R. Grilli, J. Grimshaw and A. Oxman, eds). Available in The Cochrane Library [database on disk and CDROM]. The Cochrane Collaboration, issue 1. Oxford: Update Software, 1998 [updated quarterly].

Thomson, M. A., Oxman, A. D., Haynes, R. B., et al. (1998d). Local opinion leaders to improve health professional practice and health care outcomes. In *Cochrane Collaboration on Effective Professional Practice Module of the Cochrane Database of Systematic Reviews* [updated 01 December 1997] (L. Bero, R. Grilli, J. Grimshaw and A. Oxman, eds). Available in The Cochrane Library [database on disk and CDROM]. The Cochrane Collaboration, issue 1. Oxford: Update Software, 1998 [updated quarterly].

Turner, P. and Whitfield, T. W. A. (1997). Physiotherapists' use of evidence based practice: a cross-national study. *Physiother Res Int*, **2**(1), 17–29.

Turner, P. A. and Whitfield, T. W. A. (1996). A multivariate analysis of physiotherapy clinicians' journal readership. *Physiother Theory Practice*, **12**, 221–30.

Wensing, M. and Grol, R. (1994). Single and combined strategies for implementing changes in primary care: a literature review. *Int J Qual Health Care*, **6**, 115–32.

5

Involving service users

Gill Needham and Sandy Oliver

Introduction

This chapter will ask you to consider where those people who use health services, the patients, fit into the process of evidence-based healthcare. It will focus on three areas of your professional life:

- You and your patients
- Developing policy and planning services
- Doing and using research.

To illustrate the arguments put forward in this chapter, you will be introduced to Mrs Patience and the decisions she faces when experiencing chronic low back pain. Sue, her physiotherapist, hopes to offer Mrs Patience a choice of treatments based on the best available evidence of effectiveness. You will also be asked to consider how Sue might invite Mrs Patience and other service users to work together to develop a more evidence-based physiotherapy service.

You and your patients

Consider the following scenario:

Sue is a physiotherapist in a busy department in a small district general hospital. A middle-aged woman with chronic low back pain, Mrs Patience is referred to the department by her general practitioner (GP). Like most patients, she wants to know what is wrong with her back. Why does she have a problem? What has caused it? Will she get better without help or would she do better with treatment? On the advice of friends, one of the things she has been considering is buying a transcutaneous electrical nerve stimulation (TENS) machine, which she has been told relieves pain, for use at home. She has also heard about back schools and wants to know whether this approach is likely to help her. How can Sue help her to find the information she needs and give her support while she makes up her mind?

Mrs Patience's questions will be familiar to any health professional. Typically, when people are ill, they want to know (Helman, 1984):

- What has happened? Can the symptoms and signs be recognized and given a name or identity?
- Why has it happened? Does the condition have a clear aetiology?
- Why has it happened to me? Does the illness relate to aspects of the patient such as behaviour, diet, body-build, personality or heredity?
- Why now? Is the timing of the illness significant; is progression sudden or slow?
- What would happen if nothing was done about it? What is the likely course, outcome, prognosis and danger?
- What should I do about it? What options are there for treating the condition? Should I try self-medication, consultation with friends and family, or going to see the doctor?

The last question is unlikely to be answered by simply calling on expert knowledge. It requires a decision.

How do individuals make decisions?

Making decisions is not simple. Every decision is unique. The needs and preferences of people for information, their expectations and their personality traits, all differ and influence how treatment choices are made. Most choices are not made in a rational and measured way. People draw on many sources of information which may be unreliable, and they tend to focus on aspects that fit their preconceptions. People also differ in their attitudes to choice about treatment. Sometimes they want choice, sometimes they want their carer to make the choice for them, and sometimes they want to be able to choose whether or not to be given the choice.

How information about healthcare effectiveness is structured and presented affects the way in which people understand and use it:

- The order in which information is presented
- Which types of information are presented together
- Whether messages are offered in a positive or negative framework, or both
- How probabilities are expressed
- How scales and graphs are drawn
- How the degree of certainty is implied.

These all affect how patients deal with the information they receive. They may also be influenced by the original source of the information and whether the information presented reflects their cultural background.

The patient–practitioner relationship

The majority of health decisions are taken without involving a practitioner. For example, whether to take paracetamol for a headache, or which over-the-counter preparation to buy for travel sickness, or whether to keep a child at home from school because of a bad cough. How decisions are made when someone consults a practitioner depends on the relationship between the two and how they share information and decisions (Charles et al, 1997).

Traditionally, once a health professional was consulted, it was he or she who took responsibility for the decisions, and the patient assumed the passive role of recipient of advice. The health professional acted on behalf of the patient, choosing both the treatment and how much to tell the patient about it. Whether this is seen as reassuring and paternalistic or authoritarian and coercive will depend on how the patient and the carer feel about sharing the decisions that have to be made. There are powerful arguments against this approach. People have a right to information about their own bodies and what is likely to happen to them. Furthermore, it has been known for some time that well-informed patients cope better with their treatment, experience less pain and have better outcomes than those without information (Hayward, 1975; Ley, 1988).

An alternative approach would be for the practitioner to provide information, to avoid giving advice in case such advice might bias the patient, and to provide the treatment that the patient then chooses. This approach may be seen as a respect for the autonomy of the patient. To respect the autonomy of the practitioner simultaneously, it also needs to leave the practitioner free to refer the patient elsewhere for care if he or she is unable or unwilling to provide the patient's chosen treatment.

Both approaches, however, neglect the importance of:

- Combining dialogue with support for decision-making
- The considerable variation between patients in the responsibility they wish to assume for decisions about their treatment and care
- How an individual may vary over time or when facing different decisions.

A partnership is called for in which patient and practitioner share both information and opinions and take steps to build a consensus about the preferred treatment (Charles et al, 1997). This more flexible approach encourages discussion and debate, with practitioners offering far more than information and technical skills, offering emotional support for decision-making too.

In this partnership of shared decision-making, the evidence about the effectiveness of treatments and their alternatives is made equally accessible to patient and professional and is discussed openly and on equal terms, including the gaps in knowledge and areas of uncertainty.

Health professionals need specific skills in order to share decision-making with their patients. This involves not only communication skills and knowledge of evidence and information sources but, importantly, an understanding of the complexity of individual decision-making. The practitioner needs to be aware of, and sensitive to, each individual patient's values and how these values may influence the way he or she approaches a decision. In distressing or worrying situations, the practitioner may also need emotional support. The need for this range of skills and peer support networks should first be addressed in basic training and then developed further as part of continuing professional development.

Returning to Mrs Patience. She wishes to make her own decisions about treatment, with support and advice from Sue. She wants access to all available evidence about alternative treatments in order to make her own judgements. She is also prepared to devote some time to this if necessary. Sue recognizes that her decision-making will be influenced by her wish to be active in her own care, so self-care aspects will be important here. Her social situation may also be important. She runs her own business from home, which gives her some flexibility in managing her time, but also some pressure to return to work as soon as possible. She has support from her family and is prepared to incur some costs, e.g. for a TENS machine, but is unwilling to go outside the National Health Service (NHS) for treatment.

Practice points

- Do you recognize which of your patients like to make decisions for themselves, which prefer you to make decisions on their behalf and which share information and decisions with you?
- Try offering information about treatments without necessarily choosing a treatment for a patient.
- How do you explain complex information to your patients? Do you scribble diagrams and graphs or tell them the risk of something working well and the risk of it not working well (positive and negative framing)?
- Do you explain conditions and treatments in plain English to ensure that your patients understand, then add the technical terms so they will recognize them if they hear or read them elsewhere?
- Do you ask patients for their opinions about treatments?

Users' access to information about healthcare

To support informed decision-making, patients require access to information about their treatments, preferably written in plain English. Where should they go for this kind of information? There is a vast amount of information for the public about health problems. Women's magazines, specialist health magazines and an increasing number of television and radio programmes focus on specific topics. Popular medical books are best sellers, especially those related to women's and children's health. For specific problems and treatments, the most accessible source is probably a leaflet or booklet. These are produced by a range of organizations and individuals including the pharmaceutical and medical equipment industries, support groups, medical charities, professional bodies, health authorities, trusts and individual practitioners.

Health information services

A wide variety of books and leaflets are held by Consumer Health Information Services. These are services set up specifically to deal with information requests from the public on any aspect of health, illness or health services. Some services are based in public libraries, some in shops, some in hospitals, and many are telephone services. In 1992, the Patient's Charter required each of the then 14 regional health authorities in England to make a health information service available to all their residents, giving information on common illnesses and treatments, self-help groups, health services, waiting times, keeping healthy and complaints procedures. This network of services is linked by a single freephone number. Anyone can phone 0800 665544 and be transferred to the nearest service to deal with their enquiry. There are now 26 services in England and Wales, for details of information lines in Scotland and Northern Ireland see Appendix 2.

The staff working in these services are experts in giving information. Their work can complement that of health professionals. In some areas, health professionals will refer patients to the local health information service to find information which they can then share and discuss. Alternatively, health professionals may contact the services to locate information for their clients. The services deal with a range of enquiries. Many callers ask about the nature of illness or the process of treatment and care, for example, what will happen to me, what do they do in this operation? Others, like Mrs Patience, ask questions about choices of treatments.

Support groups

Support groups play an invaluable role in giving information as well as support for their particular areas of expertise. Most national groups produce their own information, much of which is of excellent quality. The advantage they have is their knowledge of the questions that people want answered. An example of a thriving national group that Mrs Patience may find useful is the Back Pain Association. The Association has a large membership of both sufferers and practitioners, as well as a network of local branches throughout the UK. A range of information is produced: leaflets, research reports and newsletters. In addition, a helpline gives information and support to sufferers.

The Internet

An increasingly popular source of health information is the Internet, following an exponential growth in the number of households with access. Searching reveals a vast range of sources, from academic medical libraries to local support groups. While the lack of any filter or quality control must be a cause for concern, the potential of the Internet to empower individuals is considerable. Health professionals will find themselves dealing with an increasingly informed public and this will contribute to the pressure for them to keep abreast of emerging evidence.

Practitioners

Most people prefer to get information from a healthcare professional, usually the doctor, nurse or therapist who is caring for them. Many professionals rely on giving information verbally. However:

- Skills in giving information vary between health professionals
- People forget what they have been told in a consultation, especially if they are anxious
- People frequently fail to ask the questions in the consultation that afterwards they need answered
- Even if they remember what they have been told, people may find it difficult to discuss it with their family afterwards.

Practice points

Try to ensure that information given verbally is understood and remembered by:

- Reinforcing messages and checking back
- Providing notes and diagrams if no printed information is available
- Speaking to relatives or carers, as well as to patients, if appropriate
- Sending your patients elsewhere for further information
- Finding out about local information sources, e.g. Consumer Health Information Services and self-help groups.

Recognizing high-quality evidence-based information

There is clearly a need for high-quality evidence-based information produced in accessible formats, ideally to be used by patients and professionals together. Unfortunately, despite the increasing volume of patient information available, the quality is very patchy. The majority of information available about treatments tends to describe the **process**, for example, what is TENS, what will it feel like, or how they do a spinal fusion, rather than the **outcomes**, such as reduced pain or better mobility. The process is important to patients, but they need information about the outcomes too. Patients need some idea of the evidence for the effectiveness of a treatment, the benefits and risks, and the possible alternatives, including the likely outcome of no treatment, to help them make decisions.

Producing high-quality evidence-based information for your patients

The development of evidence-based patient information, regardless of format, should incorporate the following stages (Coulter, 1997):

- Determine the patients' information needs
- Systematically review the research evidence

- Decide how the material will be accessed and used
- Choose the most appropriate media
- Develop the information package.

An illustration of this process is the development and piloting of leaflets on surgery for cataracts (Buckinghamshire Health Authority and NHS Centre for Reviews and Dissemination, 1996). Two focus groups were set up: one comprised a group of patients who had undergone cataract surgery and the other a multidisciplinary group of professionals involved in eye care. The focus groups were initially asked to identify the questions that patients ask, or would like to ask, about having cataracts removed. The relevant evidence was produced by systematically reviewing the literature, and a draft leaflet was developed and returned to both focus groups for comment and amendment.

The value of a patient focus group in identifying the questions to be addressed by patient information cannot be overstated. This was illustrated in a multidisciplinary project to develop information leaflets about treatment options for women suffering from heavy periods (Buckinghamshire Health Authority, 1995). Two focus groups of sufferers were asked about their information needs on the topic. The issues raised were notably different from those expected by the project team.

At later stages of the process, a focus group can help with presentation and readability, particularly to flag up the use of technical or NHS terminology and, if appropriate, to help with the development of user-friendly glossaries.

The Centre for Health Information Quality (CHiQ)

Advice in preparing patient information is available from the national Centre for Health Information Quality. This was set up in 1997, funded by the NHS Executive, to encourage the development of evidence-based patient information and to disseminate work carried out in this area (Gann, 1997). The Centre is highlighting three equally important aspects of quality in information for patients:

1. **The evidence base**. Does it incorporate the most up-to-date evidence on the topic?
2. **The presentation**. How readable is it? Is the layout eye-catching?
3. **The user focus**. Were users involved in producing the information, to ensure that the important questions were addressed?

The principles of critical appraisal, described in Chapter 7, should be as applicable to patient information as they are to systematic reviews or reports of individual studies. To this end, a project called DISCERN was funded by the British Library Research and Development Department, to develop and pilot an assessment tool for patient literature (Charnock et al, 1997). This tool consists of a number of questions, for example, are the choices of treatment made clear, is the information unbiased? The Centre for Health Information Quality will be testing DISCERN alongside other tools for assessing information quality, including readability tests.

Interactive video programmes

Formats more sophisticated than leaflets include interactive videos, designed specifically to help patients share treatment decisions with their healthcare professionals (Darkins, 1994). These were first developed in the USA at Dartmouth Medical School and Massachusetts General Hospital. These videos allow patients to explore the evidence on the consequences of alternative treatment decisions. Since 1992, the Kings Fund has been involved in evaluating their effectiveness (Shepperd et al, 1995).

Returning once more to Mrs Patience: Sue wonders whether there is any evidence-based patient information that will help her to decide what to do next. She contacts the local Consumer Health Information Service. They supply some leaflets and a contact number for the Back Pain Association.

On Mrs Patience's next visit they discuss the information they have received: a pile of leaflets from national organizations, the local health promotion department and other sources, and a selection of popular journal articles. The leaflets are extremely practical, focusing on helping people cope. The majority are about self-care and exercise. Mrs Patience selects a couple that will help her to maintain the exercise programme that Sue has recommended.

There is, however, little information about the effectiveness of different treatments. Mrs Patience likes *The Back Book* (Royal College of General Practitioners, 1996) but unfortunately neither this nor any of the other patient information answer her question about the effectiveness of TENS. Sue looks at some useful reviews of evidence on the management of back pain: the report from the Clinical Standards Advisory Group (1994), *Clinical Guidelines for the Management of Acute Low Back Pain* (Royal College of General Practitioners, 1996) and the Cochrane Library. The Cochrane Library yields a systematic review of TENS which concludes that the treatment is effective for chronic low back pain (Gadsby and Flowerdew, 1997).

Practice points

- Do you give your patients leaflets or other information produced commercially or by support groups?
- If so, do you check the quality and the evidence base of the information?
- How do you decide what is acceptable quality for your patients?
- Do you or your department produce your own leaflets for patients?

If so:

- Do you ask patients what are the questions they want answered?
- Do you ensure that the information is based on the most up-to-date evidence?
- Do you pilot information to ensure that the language and presentation are appropriate?

Suggestion: if you are producing patient information for the first time:

- Check that you are not duplicating something already available (ask the Centre for Health Information Quality)

- Involve service users from the start, for example, organize a focus group, to find out the questions which they would like you to address
- Seek out the most up-to-date reliable evidence
- Ask your users to help you to check the readability and presentation of the information
- Pilot a leaflet with as many people as you can.

Informed patients improve practice

Developing evidence-based information for patients may have value other than informing people and helping them to make decisions about their care. Informed patients may influence practitioners to implement evidence-based practice (Freemantle et al, 1997) and eventually improve outcomes. Reviews of strategies used to change clinical practice (Davis et al, 1995; Oxman et al, 1995) include patient-mediated interventions alongside methods like educational outreach or specialist conferences, which were discussed in Chapter 4. Patient expectations undoubtedly influence the care they receive. Ill-informed patients can demand unnecessary and possibly harmful interventions. For example, most GPs are aware of the guidelines from the Royal College of Radiologists (1993) which recommend that lumbar X-rays should not be performed routinely for back pain, but many admit that they nevertheless request them because patients expect and demand them. Alternatively, patients may request care that is known to be effective, but which is not always available.

Developing policy and planning services

Mrs Patience's request for information about TENS comes at an opportune moment for Sue and her department. The Head of Therapy Services has been made aware of the Cochrane review of TENS and feels that this new evidence may well support the case for developing a new service within the department, a TENS machine loan service for back pain sufferers. Sue is asked to prepare a case of need, for submission to the health authority.

Commissioners (primary care groups and health authorities) need to ensure that the services they purchase will meet the needs of local people. In making a decision about a service, they need to obtain and weigh up the best possible evidence about effectiveness, cost and human resource implications, as well as local clinical experience, the views of the public and the experience of patients. Trusts or individual services or departments looking at service development are faced with the same challenge.

While the involvement of patients in decisions about their personal care is widely accepted, far fewer health professionals have experience of working in partnership with patients in the planning and monitoring of services. This situation is, however, gradually changing. A trust board, a rehabilitation team or a therapy department considering a new service may choose to involve users in this process. Service users may take the initiative themselves and ask to meet professionals and service managers. Rather than waiting for pressures from outside, health professionals may invite patients to work with them in planning, monitoring and evaluating services because they have valuable insights arising from their experiences as service users. Local user or patient groups have an important role here because they have access to a wide range of views and experiences and may have easier access to groups, such as carers of housebound or older people.

Formal approaches to user involvement

Methods of ascertaining public and patient or user views and their experience are becoming increasingly sophisticated. The choice of method will depend on the nature and size of the issue being explored.

Patient satisfaction surveys

Whether carried out by post, telephone or brief encounters in waiting rooms, these have been perceived as the standard method over recent years for finding out patients' views on care and services.

Questionnaires can be useful for collecting data on simple and well-defined issues. Their design should be carefully planned and piloted to ensure that they provide:

- The required data
- Data that can be analysed and used
- An unbiased response.

Investing additional time interviewing people can elicit important qualitative insights and may be particularly helpful for marginalized service users (Thomas, undated).

Meetings, stakeholder conferences and focus groups

These methods have the distinct advantage of offering more time for thought and discussion. Public meetings are often poorly organized and may (sometimes rightly) be perceived as public relations exercises rather than genuine attempts to identify public views and concerns. Stakeholder conferences can be very powerful but are expensive and require considerable skills to organize and facilitate. In Buckinghamshire, for example, in 1996 all key stakeholders in services for cancer patients (all provider trusts, primary care, patient groups, community health councils) attended such a conference, facilitated by the Office of Public Management, to try to identify the way forward for cancer care.

Focus groups may also require independent facilitation to protect their neutrality. They are an excellent way of generating ideas, however, for instance when developing patient-focused standards for a service.

Citizens' juries

Pioneering attempts to elicit public preferences are now criticized for asking the public to make uninformed decisions. For instance, when people in Hackney (Bowling et al, 1993) were asked to prioritize different health services, they were not given information about the frequency of conditions or effectiveness of the treatments and care involved, and were therefore working on the basis of values alone.

An approach that seeks to address this particular criticism is the citizens' jury, in which a jury of local people addresses a question, hears evidence from expert witnesses, deliberates and then makes recommendations to the appropriate decision making body. In Buckinghamshire, a citizens' jury was used to involve local people in determining the way in which services for people with back pain should be developed (Friend, 1997). The jury focused particularly on whether the services of osteopaths and chiropractors should be available within the NHS for people with back pain. The jury's role was to study the evidence of effectiveness and weigh this up with the complex array of information about costs, professional views and personal experience presented to it. Over a period of $4\frac{1}{2}$ days, the jury heard evidence about the epidemiology of back pain, the latest evidence from systematic reviews about the clinical effectiveness of a range of back pain treatments (Evans and Richards, 1996; Van Tulder et al, 1996), the views and experience of a GP, an orthopaedic surgeon, an osteopath, a chiropractor and a physiotherapist, and the personal experiences of back pain sufferers. They also learned about the financial implications for both purchasers and trusts of making service changes. After deliberation, they recommended moving towards specialist back pain clinics with multidisciplinary staff teams, including osteopaths and chiropractors, as well as physiotherapists.

A similar initiative in Italy involved consumers in presenting evidence as well as judging its value for policy development (Working Group on Socio-Psychological Implications of Follow-up, 1995).

Critically appraising the evidence together

Innovative ways of sharing information about effectiveness and decisions about care rest on the close scrutiny of the evidence. Critically appraising a report with a multidisciplinary group informs the participants about evidence of effectiveness and is a useful way of unearthing important questions (Oliver, 1996).

The Critical Appraisal Skills Programme's experience of working with community health councils, consumer health information services (Milne and Oliver, 1996), and maternity service liaison committees (Crowe, 1997) shows that critical appraisal workshops enable constructive discussion between people with diverse backgrounds and perspectives, including service users. Clearly, multidisciplinary learning, despite its challenges, could pay dividends in working relationships.

Developing clinical guidelines

Locally developed (or nationally developed and locally adapted) clinical guidelines can play an important role in introducing evidence-based practice, as described in Chapter 8, but these should involve service users early in the development stage. The knowledge and experience of service users are important parts of the evidence required, for example their experience of the illness, the treatment they received and the availability of services. In Australia (Bastian, 1996) a national body ensures user involvement in all guideline development.

Practice points

- What is your experience of involving users/patients in developing your service?
- Have you carried out any patient satisfaction surveys?
- Have you ever attended any public meetings organized by your trust or department to consult users?
- Do you work with any local patient groups?
- Do you involve users informally in policy development and planning?
- Do you involve users in developing clinical guidelines?

If the answer to any of these is yes, what have you learned from the experience?

Barriers and solutions

Developing services based on research evidence is an imprecise task. The information available may not be complete and some may be considered more valuable than others. Differences in values and perspectives become most readily apparent when managers, practitioners and users all have a voice.

Playing a part in service planning is a real challenge for users. They need to understand technical language, how the health service is organized and how committees function. They need communication, advocacy and organizational skills. They would like to feel more confident and be more assertive. Health professionals may also find sharing the planning a challenge for other reasons. Multidisciplinary teamwork is becoming more common within the NHS but not necessarily more successful with its 'inherent professional hierarchies... and mutual ignorance of different professionals' skills and modus operandi [which means] that skilled leadership and adequate time are required to ensure that all panel members are actively involved... These issues become more important when patients are involved... the asymmetry of information, the perceived status of healthcare professionals and the technical discussions... make it difficult for patients to contribute actively' (Grimshaw et al, 1995).

One solution has been to allow each different type of patient, carer and health professional a separate forum for discussion with a formal method for recording their views and suggestions (Hare et al, 1992). However, this leaves the task of trying to reconcile differences between the groups. It may be wise in the event of any disagreements, however issues views have been elicited, for decision-makers to be explicit about how they responded to information generated by consultation with users with which they did not agree (Martin and Evans, 1993).

Sue's task is to prepare a case of need for a new TENS service. While she has some evidence of clinical effectiveness from the Cochrane review and some information about costs, she feels that the case would be better informed still by collecting the views and experience of some users of TENS. In order to elicit these she decides to convene a patient focus group. At the same time she requires some views from a wider group of back pain sufferers (TENS users and non-TENS users) to see how TENS is rated in the context of other aspects of the service. She contacts the local back pain group and they help her to carry out a simple questionnaire survey. The group's involvement in the questionnaire design is crucial in ensuring that the right questions are asked, and that the language and presentation are user-friendly. Having gathered her evidence in this way and drafted her proposal, she contacts the public health department of the local health authority and discovers that members of the department are about to convene a meeting of a multidisciplinary group of professionals and patients to develop local clinical guidelines for the management of low back pain. She is invited to join the group which, on her suggestion, works together to critically appraise the Cochrane review of TENS (Gadsby and Flowerdew, 1997). The group decides that the evidence from the review and from Sue's focus group and patient survey warrants taking the proposal forward. The Head of Therapy is delighted.

Practice points

- Be proactive in involving users in policy and planning
- Discuss any concerns about user involvement with your colleagues and agree to share learning as you go along
- Organize an informal group of your patients to critically appraise a new piece of evidence
- Set up a focus group to help you to develop a series of questions to ask in a patient satisfaction survey
- Invite one or two users to attend a departmental meeting to join in the discussion and contribute their views of the service
- Identify and join local multidisciplinary groups.

Doing and using research

Research from the patients' perspective

Appraising reviews from a patient's viewpoint may reveal that some questions are not satisfied with answers at all, even poor-quality answers. For instance, the Cochrane systematic review of TENS (Gadsby and Flowerdew, 1997) suggests that TENS appears to reduce pain and improve the range of movement in people with chronic low back pain. However, it does not provide information about how TENS fares when compared with other treatments, or when used simultaneously with other treatments, or how long improvements can be expected to last. Neither does it explain whether TENS improves patients' ability to cope with their routine daily tasks, hastens their return to work, or enhances their general well-being.

At present, as is often the case, Mrs Patience can only be partially informed before making her decision. Future patients may be better informed by new, rigorous studies, where patients' questions are addressed simultaneously with professionals' questions. Involving patients or people with experience of particular clinical services, or the potential to call on these, helps to focus the design of new studies.

Patients contribute important perceptions about health-related behaviour, observations about health services, explanations of lay values and priorities, skills in representing their peers, or their fresh insights and strong motivation. They may help to recruit participants to trials or to develop information to invite patients' consent to participate. Alternatively, user groups may take the initiative and undertake their own research, or commission researchers to work under their direction.

Measuring the benefits of, for example, physiotherapy, is a challenging task, and is even more so if the conclusions of research are to inform patients. Although physiotherapists are familiar with exercise regimes that aim to help patients regain mobility, balance and strength while reducing pain, **measuring** changes in mobility, balance and strength is not easy. In a study that was trying to help patients with osteoarthritis of the knee, their progress was measured with scales designed to detect changes in pain, medication, physical activity and their overall physical, mental and social well-being (or quality of life), as well as the distance they could walk. While a randomized controlled trial employing these scales enabled researchers to detect the effectiveness of an exercise programme, the details reported in the paper were insufficient to describe the severity of symptoms experienced by patients in the trial, or which symptoms were alleviated and to what degree (Kovar et al, 1992). Meaningful information to patients was therefore limited. Recording participants' experiences alongside quantitative data may illustrate effectiveness better.

Consumers' contributions to research

When planning research, whether the questions that need addressing relate to decisions about individual care or to planning and monitoring services, there are opportunities to bring service users' perspectives to the measurement of outcomes (UK Clearing House on Health Outcomes, 1996). This requires asking what outcomes are important to patients:

- How can they be measured to reflect patients' priorities?
- In the patients' view, what are the most appropriate times for measuring outcomes?
- How can outcome measures inform decisions about individual care, service evaluation, audit and planning?

When important outcomes are missing, an evaluation may be misleading. If readmission to hospital is an outcome measure for assessing effectiveness of rehabilitation programmes following hip fracture, is this a good outcome or a poor outcome? Researchers who recognize that this interpretation may differ between patients and their families or carers might include carer burden or stress in their full array of outcome measures.

Developing measures from the user perspective requires listening to users to either identify key outcomes or construct composite scales that address a range of issues important to patients. For instance, the Carer Satisfaction Questionnaire (Pound and Gompertz, 1993) was designed from interviews with carers and a search of published reports. In-depth interviews were conducted with six carers. The subsequent draft questionnaire was then piloted and a final version developed. The questionnaire covers two key areas of carer need, information provision and adequacy of support. It could be used to monitor the effects of different levels and types of support and services provided, for example, to stroke patients after discharge from hospital.

Consumers' own research

Service users not only bring useful perspectives to individual research projects, but they may also raise awareness of new areas for study. Many self-help groups explore issues that are important to people using the health services. This may offer important insights to health professionals about the difficulties that patients face, how patients view their care, their priorities and their suggestions for improving care at home, in the voluntary sector and within the NHS. Some user-led research focuses not on how to cure health problems, but on the information and support that service users, their families and carers, need while they try to cope with health problems related to, for example, pregnancy and childbirth, childhood problems, poverty and cancer (Oliver and Buchanan, 1997). Most user-led research has been funded by the user organizations themselves, although some has been commissioned by health authorities who saw user groups as having the most appropriate experience for this kind of investigation.

Collaborative research

If a variety of research reports address the same question of effectiveness, discussing their findings may be easier if they are gathered together in a systematic review. People working within the Cochrane Collaboration to review the literature in this way are encouraged to involve consumers in their work. They are invited to suggest and prioritize questions for review (for example, which interventions should be compared among which population of people and with what outcomes), to find studies, and to comment on the findings and offer constructive criticism.

Practice points

- Have you been involved in research? If so, were service users involved too?
- Have self-help groups undertaken research relevant to your physiotherapy patients?

Some months later Sue is reminded of Mrs Patience and the inadequacy of information available to help her decision making, when she sees a conference advertised about involving service users in all healthcare decisions. The keynote presentation is to be joint between an officer of a royal college and a volunteer from a self-help group, describing how they brought together patients, carers, practitioners, purchasers and provider managers to scrutinize the evidence, develop practice guidelines and prepare evidence-based patient information.

Summary

By sharing information with their patients, health professionals help patients to cope better with treatments, experience less pain and achieve better outcomes (Hayward, 1975; Ley, 1988). Sharing decisions, as well as information, allows the choice of treatment to reflect individual patients' concerns and lifestyles. Involving patients in planning can make services more relevant to their needs by drawing on their insights and understanding. The practical task of preparing information for patients leads to a better product if it has been carried out in partnership with patients or self help groups who understand the questions that patients ask and are able to comment on the clarity of patient information.

Evidence-based patient choice is a new and developing area. Incorporating the user perspective in all aspects of the evidence-based healthcare agenda, rather than treating it as an optional extra, will be much more effective. Waiting until nearing the end of a project to invite user comment or finalize patient information will merely serve to highlight the discrepancies between users' and professionals' perspectives without offering opportunities to address them constructively. Far better is to involve users from the beginning and build good working relationships to integrate the different perspectives.

Prompted by her experience of caring for Mrs Patience, Sue attends the conference about involving service users in all healthcare decision-making. This is a forum for meeting potential partners, for discussing ways of working together, for hearing how patients have contributed to new research, and for Sue to tell her story about involving patients in developing a new physiotherapy service. As a result of the conference, she also volunteers to join a colleague and members of self-help groups who are already peer reviewing research of physiotherapy treatments within the Cochrane Collaboration.

Further reading

Barker, J., Bullen, M. and de Ville, J. (1997). *Reference Manual for Public Involvement*. Bromley Health Authority.

Dunning, M., Needham, G. and Weston, S. (eds) (1997). *But Will It Work, Doctor?* Report of a second 'But will it work, doctor?' conference. Consumer Health Information Consortium.

Hamilton Gurney, B. (1994). *Public Participation in Health Care*. Health Services Research Group, University of Cambridge.

Stewart, J., Kendall, E. and Coote, A. (1995). Citizens' Juries. Institute for Public Policy Research.

References

Bastian, H. (1996). Raising the standard: practice guidelines and consumer participation. *Int J Qual Health Care*, **8**(5), 485–90.

Bowling, A., Jacobson, B. and Southgate, L. (1993). Explorations in consultation of the public and health professionals on priority setting in an inner London health district. *Soc Sci Med*, **37**, 851–57.

Buckinghamshire Health Authority and the NHS Centre for Reviews and Dissemination (1996). *Cataract: Information for Patients*. Buckinghamshire Health Authority.

Buckinghamshire Health Authority (1995). *Heavy Periods – You Can Get Help*. Buckinghamshire Health Authority.

Charles, C., Gafni, A. and Whelan, T. (1997). Shared decision-making in the medical encounter: what does it mean? *Soc Sci Med*, **44**, 681–92.

Charnock, D., Shepperd, S, Needham, G., et al. (1997). *DISCERN: Developing an Assessment Instrument for the Critical Appraisal of Written Consumer Health Information*. 2nd International Conference Scientific Basis of Health Services, Amsterdam.

Clinical Standards Advisory Group (1994). *Back Pain: Report of a CSAG Committee on Back Pain*. HMSO.

Coulter, A. (1997). Developing evidence-based patient information. In *But Will It Work, Doctor?* Report of a second 'But will it work, doctor?' conference. (M. Dunning, G. Needham and S. Weston, eds) pp. 30–3, Consumer Health Information Consortium.

Crowe, S. (1997). CASP for MSLCs: a project enabling maternity service liaison committees to develop an evidence based approach to Changing Childbirth. Critical Appraisal Skills Programme, Oxford Institute of Health Sciences.

Darkins, A. (1994). Sharing decision-making with patients. In *But Will It Work, Doctor?* Report of a conference about involving users of health services in outcomes research (M. Dunning and G. Needham, eds) pp. 9–11, Consumer Health Information Consortium.

Davis, D. A., Thomson, M. A., Oxman, A. D. and Haynes, R. B. (1995). Changing physician performance: a systematic review of the effect of continuing medical education strategies. *JAMA*, **274**(9), 700–5.

Evans, G. and Richards, S. (1996). *Low Back Pain: An Evaluation of Therapeutic Interventions*. Health Care Evaluation Unit, University of Bristol.

Freemantle, N., Harvey, E. L., Wolf, F., et al. (1998). Printed educational materials to improve the behaviour of health care professionals and patient outcomes. In *Cochrane Collaboration on Effective Professional Practice Module of the Cochrane Database of Systematic Reviews* [updated 01 December 1997] (L. Bero, R. Grilli, J. Grimshaw and A. Oxman, eds) Available in The Cochrane Library [database on disk and CDROM]. The Cochrane Collaboration, Issue 1. Oxford: Update Software, 1998. [updated quarterly].

Friend, B. (1997). Physiotherapy services on trial. *Physiother Frontline*, **3**(6), 12.

Gadsby, J. G. and Flowerdew, M. W. (1997). The effectiveness of transcutaneous electrical nerve stimulation (TENS) and acupuncture-like transcutaneous electrical nerve stimulation (ALTENS) in the treatment of patients with chronic low back pain. In *Back Review Group for Spinal Module of The Cochrane Database of Systematic Reviews* [updated 02 December 1997]. (C. Bombardier, A. Nachemson, R. Deyo, et al, eds) Available in The Cochrane Library [database on disk and CDROM]. The Cochrane Collaboration, Issue 1. Oxford: Update Software, [updated quarterly].

Gann, R. (1997). Healthy questions. *Nursing Times*, **93**(14), 14.

Grimshaw, J., Eccles, M. and Russell, I. (1995). Developing clinically valid practice guidelines. *J Eval Clin Pract*, **1**(1), 37–48.

Hare, T., Spencer, J., Gallagher, M. et al. (1992). Diabetes care: who are the experts? *Qual Health Care*, **1**, 219–24.

Hayward, J. (1975). *Information: A Prescription Against Pain*. Royal College of Nursing.

Helman, C. (1984). *Culture, Health and Illness*. Wright.

Kovar, P. A., Allegrandte, J. P., MacKenzie, R., et al. (1992). Supervized fitness walking in patients with osteoarthritis of the knee. A randomized controlled trial. *Ann Intern Med*, **116**, 529–34.

Ley, P. (1988). *Communicating With Patients*. Croom Helm.

Martin, M. and Evans, M. (1993). *Framework for Public Involvement*. East Anglia Regional Health Authority.

Milne, R. and Oliver, S. (1996). Evidence-based consumer health information: developing teaching in critical appraisal skills. *Int J Qual Health Care*, **8**(5), 439–45.

Oliver, S. (1996). Exploring lay perspectives on questions of effectiveness. In *Non-random Reflections on Health Services* (A. Maynard and I. Chalmers, eds) pp. 272–91, BMJ Publishing Group.

Oliver, S. and Buchanan, P. (1997). *Examples of Lay Involvement in Health Research. Report to the Standing Advisory Group on Consumer Involvement in the Research and Development Programme*. Social Science Research Unit, London University Institute of Education.

Oxman, A. D., Thomson, M. A., Davis, D. A. and Haynes, R. B. (1995). No magic bullets: a systematic review of 102 trials of interventions to improve professional practice. *Can Med Assoc J*, **153**(10), 1423–31.

Pound, P. and Gompertz, E. S. (1993). Development and results of a questionnaire to measure carer satisfaction after stroke. *J Epidemiol Community Health*, **4**(6), 500–5.

Royal College of General Practitioners (1996). *Clinical Guidelines for the Management of Acute Low Back Pain*. Royal College of General Practitioners.

Royal College of General Practitioners (1996). *The Back Book*. HMSO.

Royal College of Radiologists (1993). *Making the Best Use of a Department of Clinical Radiology: Guidelines for Doctors*. Royal College of Radiologists.

Shepperd, S., Coulter, A. and Farmer, A. (1995). Using interactive videos in general practice to inform patients about treatment choices: a pilot study. *Fam Pract*, **12**, 443–7.

Thomas, B. W. (undated). *Consulting Consumers in the NHS: A Guideline Study. Services for Elderly People with Dementia Living at Home*. National Consumer Council.

UK Clearing House on Health Outcomes (1996). *Outcomes for the Patient and Carer.* Outcomes briefing 8. Nuffield Institute for Health.

Van Tulder, M. W., Koes, B. W. and Bouter, L. M. (1996). *Low Back Pain in Primary Care.* EMGO Institute.

Working Group on Socio-Psychological Implications of Follow-up (1995). The patients' point of view: results of the working group on socio-psychological implications of follow-up. *Ann Oncol*, **6**(suppl 2), S65–8.

Developing and Applying Skills

Evidence-based healthcare uses a number of steps to move from questions through to action and evaluation of the outcome. This may require the development of new skills, such as literature searching and critical appraisal. These should be seen as adjuncts to your established skills, in practice or management. They will assist you to become a more effective decision-maker and facilitator of change, irrespective of your role within healthcare delivery or workplace setting.

Tools and mechanisms for using evidence in practice and evaluating its impact are in existence. You need to become more familiar with them if they are to be used to good effect and lead to improvements in healthcare. Some of these initiatives are at a national level and it can be difficult to see how they can be adapted to local circumstances. The following chapters are designed to give you the confidence to help you do just that.

6

Finding the evidence

Andrew Booth and Bruce Madge

A clinical scenario is the starting point for evidence-based healthcare. Consider the following example:

Clinical scenario

A 35-year-old man is recovering from surgery after injuring his hand while cleaning the blades of his lawnmower. He holds a managerial position with a local manufacturer, working to some very immediate deadlines, and his injury could not have come at a worse time. He needs his hand to be fully functioning but is concerned that the time he may have to spend in rehabilitation would have a negative effect on his business. You believe that he would best achieve a favourable outcome through early physiotherapy management of his hand, but you need to convince him that such an investment of his time is likely to prove effective. You decide to search for evidence on the benefits of early as opposed to late intervention in rehabilitation following hand surgery.

Defining your question

Unlike academic assignments in further and higher education, which often emphasize the **process** of information gathering, the above situation focuses on the **outcome**. Will the information that you retrieve help you, and your patient, to make the right treatment choice? Three key factors will help to determine the right treatment choice for this patient (Sackett et al, 1996):

1. The perceptions and aspirations of the patient
2. Your own clinical expertise
3. Evidence derived from published research (the focus of this particular chapter).

   Usually you will take the results from a study population and then decide the extent to which they can be applied to an individual patient. Once you have demonstrated the success of an intervention with an individual patient, you will consider whether this treatment might be offered to all similar patients in the future. When, and only when, you have brought the three key factors together, in the specific instance, can you start to address the wider question; 'Given that this treatment seems likely to prove beneficial in this particular patient what are the chances that it is also applicable to a larger population?' (Guyatt et al, 1994).

The bringing together of the patient's perspective, the practitioner's expertise and the research-derived evidence has two main implications for your search of the literature:

1. It is of paramount importance to identify the exact clinical question that you are trying to answer.
2. It places a requirement that you identify the best available evidence for this question in terms of its validity, reliability and appropriateness.

From the above scenario you will see that you already have a fair amount of detail on this particular problem. You have:

- A **patient** or **population**: a 35-year-old man, not a manual worker, with a hand injury that has undergone surgical repair
- An **intervention**: early physiotherapy management of the hand
- An **outcome**: full restoration of function
- A **comparison**: other forms of physiotherapy management, probably of later commencement and possibly of longer duration.

Advocates of evidence-based healthcare refer to these four elements as the **anatomy** of a clinical question (Richardson et al, 1995). This is a way of breaking down a clinical problem into a question that can be answered. If you use this anatomy it will help you either to be more clear about the question you are trying to answer or to identify elements that are of particular importance:

- What does the patient understand by full restoration of function?
- How do I define early physiotherapy?
- What alternative interventions or treatments are available?
- In which populations is this treatment particularly effective?

Referring to the earlier scenario, you can see that there is a lack of clarity in the nature of the hand injury and the type of surgery undergone in order to repair it. This could hinder your search for appropriate evidence.

Once you have broken down the available information into the four elements of the anatomy, you can use this to brainstorm alternative phrases or concepts that may be used to describe your topic, as shown in Table 6.1.

An **exposure** is where something *happens* to someone where it is not a planned occurrence, e.g. an adverse effect or an accidental fall. An **intervention**, in contrast, is a planned course of action such as surgery, drug therapy or acupuncture. A focused question may be, for example, 'In adult gardeners (population) what are the main types of accidental injury (exposure) requiring hospitalization (outcome)?'.

This brainstorming process may help you to identify key phrases, or potential subject terms, that will lead you to retrieve relevant articles.

Table 6.1 Phrasing the topic

Patient or population	Intervention or exposure		Outcome		Comparison
Adult	Early management		Mobility		Time factors
Male					
Manager	Early physiotherapy	*and*	Restoring function	*and*	Late physiotherapy
Gardener					
Hand surgery					
Hand injury(ies)					
Gardening					
Injury					

The story is told of a tourist who is driving through the countryside and stops to ask the way of a country yokel. 'Excuse me, but can you give me directions as to how to get to Barchester?' The yokel thinks long and hard and then answers, 'Well, if I was going to Barchester I wouldn't start from here'. Many searches for evidence prove unsuccessful, not because of limitations in the resources available to satisfy them, but because one has lost sight of the originating question. This is seen most often in the way that a finely focused patient-based scenario may become transformed into a bland database request such as, rehabilitation of hand injuries, human studies only, English articles only, from 1991–1997.

Steps to find the evidence

The consequences of a lack of attention to detail in defining your question may be mirrored at other stages of the process of finding the evidence (Figure 6.1). Avoid this by:

- Selecting the libraries that are most likely to yield a fruitful search
- Choosing the databases that are most appropriate for a particular topic
- Devising a search strategy to retrieve relevant items from these databases (Booth, 1996).

Just as you would not subject all your patients to the same regime, regardless of site or severity of their injury, you should not assume that the same course of information seeking will be similarly rewarding for any two clinical questions. You will find that, even if you have become proficient in finding evidence for yourself, a librarian will often be able to advise you on alternative sources, resources or search strategies. Nevertheless, it will be helpful to have a basic **toolkit** of information skills and expertise that you can adapt as circumstances require.

Step 1 of this finding-the-evidence process has already been dealt with. In step 2, **selecting the appropriate libraries** for your problem, you will need to consider the following questions:

- Is your question clinical, professional, managerial or research-based?
- Does it only concern your profession or are other professionals involved?

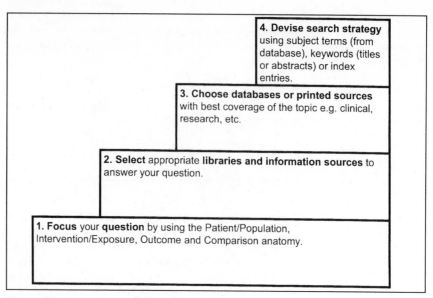

Figure 6.1 Four steps to finding the evidence.

- Is your question at a basic, intermediate or advanced level?
- Could your question be handled by an intermediary or will you have to do it yourself?
- How much time, money and effort are you prepared to spend in answering the question?

Your answer to these questions will determine whether you choose your local medical library, an information service such as that of the Chartered Society of Physiotherapy, a management collection such as that provided by the King's Fund, or a research collection held by an academic body or specialist research organization. It will also determine how much support you will require from an information professional or other intermediary, and whether you will be able to access specialist collections in person or via a telephone enquiry service.

Three useful guides to libraries that may help in your decision are:

1. the *ASLIB Directory of Information Sources in the United Kingdom* (Reynard and Reynard, 1996);
2. the British Library's *Guide to Libraries and Information Sources in Medicine and Health Care* (Dale, 1997);
3. the Chartered Society of Physiotherapy's *Introduction to Research* (Bury, 1996), with its chapter 'Literature searching: where to go and what to look for'.

With regard to step 3, the **choice of appropriate databases or printed sources**, you will have to consider the following issues:

- Is this question a current issue or is it likely to have been covered extensively in the literature?

- Is the scope of your question limited to a British context and/or to a specific discipline?
- Are the information sources easy to use and/or is assistance and support available?
- Are the sources (e.g. databases) accessible to you as an end user or will the searching have to be carried out by an intermediary?
- Are there charges associated with accessing the databases or subsequently with printing or downloading references?

Your decisions about these issues may determine whether you use a current awareness service, such as the British Library's Current Awareness Topics Services, or concentrate on sources that cover several decades. The questions will assist you in your choice between predominantly North American databases, such as MEDLINE, or those with a UK focus, such as DHSS-Data and between those covering clinical, social sciences or management topics. They may also help your choice between different formats of the same or related data: CD-ROM, online, printed or Internet. You may also encounter differences between libraries in their charging policies, even for the same database.

Finally step 4, the process of **devising the search strategy**, may be informed by the following considerations:

- Is there an established vocabulary or terminology associated with your question?
- How good is the indexing of the database at conveying your precise topic?
- Will your search be limited by language, study design or type of material?
- Do the databases that you have chosen have facilities to suggest or map your terms to approved subject terms?
- What is the relationship between the different concepts that comprise your question?

Many of these issues will be illustrated by the sample search strategies described later in this chapter.

Role of libraries

A library has a responsibility to its users to provide **relevant**, **timely** and **accurate** information. Its broad coverage, which far exceeds the scope and depth of any personal reprint collection, aims to anticipate the range of clinical problems that you may encounter. Its journal collection, with its steady stream of new and updated research, seeks to ensure access to *state-of-the-art* information in key topic areas. The cycles of revision for textbooks and the flow of debate and correspondence in clinical journals are mechanisms that aspire to accuracy. However, all these features of libraries have their limitations. With more than two million articles published annually in over 20 000 journals (Mulrow, 1994), any individual library can house only a fraction of the available literature. They are therefore dependent on access to bibliographic databases, for details of articles, and inter-library networks for delivery of items not in stock. The journal articles, of which less than 1 per cent are believed to assist in making clinical decisions (Haynes et al, 1994), are written in a manner that has been described as more a *meander* than an agenda for action (Greer, 1987). Textbooks, even when regularly updated, may take up to 3 years to produce and more than 10 years to incorporate the findings of clinically important research (Antman et al, 1992).

Evidence-based healthcare attempts to tackle these limitations in three different, yet related, ways by:

- Identifying, and in some cases providing access to, clinically significant research
- Developing techniques and products that appraise the content and context of such research
- Providing systematic overviews (or reviews) that attempt to bring together and synthesize the results of research and to highlight a clinical **bottomline**.

Foremost in activities to synthesize the research, within the UK, are two specialist information centres funded under the NHS Research and Development (R&D) Information Systems Strategy (Sheldon and Chalmers, 1994); the UK Cochrane Centre and the NHS Centre for Reviews and Dissemination.

Specialist information centres

The **Cochrane Collaboration** is an international network of healthcare professionals, researchers and consumers who prepare, maintain and disseminate systematic reviews. Collaborative **review groups** focus on a particular health problem, e.g. stroke or schizophrenia, or a particular clinical speciality, e.g. vascular surgery. Within each review group, an editorial group helps to ensure that reviews are prepared to a uniform high standard. Broader interest groups, called **fields**, seek to identify randomized controlled trials in their areas. For example, a rehabilitation and related therapies field, coordinated through the University of Maastricht, is attempting to identify trials by searching bibliographic databases and hand-searching through key journals.

Within the major countries that participate in the Cochrane Collaboration there are a number of **Cochrane Centres** that coordinate and support both the identification of trials and the production of reviews. The UK Cochrane Centre in Oxford is funded, under the NHS R&D Strategy, to provide a focus for these activities within the UK (Lefebvre, 1994). The activities of this centre and others located in countries such as Australia, Canada, France, Germany and the USA, are reflected in the production of the **Cochrane Library**, which is described in greater detail elsewhere in this chapter.

Whereas the UK Cochrane Centre is driven by the commitment and energies of individual volunteer researchers in a bottom-up approach, its sister organization, the **NHS Centre for Reviews and Dissemination** at the University of York, seeks to address an agenda identified by national and strategic priorities. Formed in January 1994, it has two main aims:

1. To increase the research-based information available to the NHS, particularly on the effectiveness and cost-effectiveness of healthcare interventions.
2. To disseminate the information effectively in a targeted way to the relevant professionals in the NHS and to consumers of its services.

The Centre for Reviews and Dissemination uses a number of methods to disseminate the reviews that it has either identified, commissioned or produced. The first of these is a **Database of Abstracts of Reviews of Effectiveness (DARE)**, available as part of the Cochrane Library or via modem or the Internet. A companion database, the **NHS Economic Evaluations Database (NEED)** focuses on cost-effectiveness studies and is available via modem or the Internet. More traditional means include a published report series, a series of topical bulletins entitled *Effective Health Care* and short four-page digests under the banner *Effectiveness Matters*. Although only a few of these items are specifically relevant to therapists, such as bulletins on stroke rehabilitation, accidental falls among elderly people and clinical guidelines, they are all serving to increase the patchwork coverage on the effectiveness of healthcare interventions. The telnet address for the DARE and NEED databases is [nhscrd.york.ac.uk] (the user ID and password are both crduser).The Web pages are at [http://www.york.ac.uk/inst/crd/welcome.htm].

Although primarily funded to be producers and compilers of research evidence, both the UK Cochrane Centre and the NHS Centre for Reviews and Dissemination offer an enquiry service that will direct callers to appropriate national and regional resources. A further enquiry service, which is also centrally funded, is the **National Centre for Clinical Audit** (Smith, 1996). This exists to support any of your information needs associated with the clinical audit process, from the setting of standards to the monitoring and evaluation of clinical effectiveness.

Information resources

There are two principal strategies for finding the evidence. Both pre-suppose that you have focused your clinical question appropriately (step 1). Strategy A is to use the traditional, more established databases (e.g. MEDLINE, AMED, ASSIA, EMBASE, CINAHL) to conduct a comprehensive search of the literature. Having retrieved relevant subject-based articles, you attempt to appraise them for value (see Chapter 7), filtering out the less useful research studies. Strategy B is to use selective specialist databases (e.g. Cochrane Library, DARE, NEED, Best Evidence) that only accept articles that meet a minimum entry standard (Booth, 1997). These studies have often been evaluated, or even fully appraised, before they are included on the specialist databases. Both approaches have their merits and these have been summarized in Table 6.2, adapted from Entwistle and colleagues (1996).

Strategy A: general databases

MEDLINE

MEDLINE is the world's largest and most popular medical database. The printed version started by John Shaw Billings in the 1870s was, and still is, produced by the United States' National Library of Medicine (NLM) in Washington DC. The database was computerized in 1966 and called MEDLINE. Currently the NLM is mounting a database called **OldMedline** which covers 1964 and 1965. Coverage of MEDLINE concentrates on peer-reviewed, predominantly American journals and, as such, it misses much of the European literature. The NLM indexes about 3700 journals out of a total of 20 000 current biomedical journals. This number tends to be static, with some titles added and some dropped each year. The popularity of MEDLINE means that you are likely to find easy access to the database in nearly all medical libraries. MEDLINE uses a controlled indexing thesaurus, called **MeSH** (Medical Subject Headings), which allows for very specific indexing and searching.

Table 6.2 Strategies for finding the evidence

STRATEGY A General databases	STRATEGY B Specialist databases
Generally available access to MEDLINE, etc.	Specialized sources, perhaps only available in specialist libraries
Generic MEDLINE skills need to be supplemented by searches for particular study designs	Multiplicity of sources with different languages and interfaces
Follow-up requirement for access to wide range of literature with no guarantees of quality	Often include access to either full text or structured abstracts allowing instant relevance judgements
User must possess full critical appraisal skills in addition to judging relevance	User must still judge relevance but appraisal has already been completed
Specialist medical terminology may prove an obstacle to interpretation	Interpretation may be provided as part of the appraisal
Broad on coverage, thin on quality assurance	Patchy on coverage but detailed in assessment

EMBASE

EMBASE, considered by some to be the European equivalent of MEDLINE, is produced by Elsevier Science in The Netherlands. It is certainly more European than MEDLINE and has specialized in pharmacological effects of drugs and chemicals. It claims to be more current than MEDLINE, but is only available back to 1974. It indexes around 3500 journals and 65 per cent of articles have full author abstracts. EMBASE, like MEDLINE, has its own thesaurus, called **EMTREE**.

AMED

AMED is the Allied and Alternative Medicine database produced by the British Library Health Care Information Service and contains bibliographic references since 1985. The database includes references on alternative medicine, physiotherapy, occupational therapy, palliative care, rehabilitation medicine and podiatry. It currently indexes around 400 journals. The thesaurus is a modified form of the NLM's MeSH headings.

CINAHL

CINAHL (Cumulated Index to Nursing and Allied Health Literature) is, as its name suggests, a nursing and allied health database produced by CINAHL Information Systems in California. Again it has a slight American bias and uses a modified MeSH thesaurus for indexing and searching. Thirty-five per cent of articles are on allied health disciplines and coverage includes around 600 journals dating from 1983. Forty-three therapy journals are covered in CINAHL, including *Dutch Journal of Physiotherapy*, *Journal of Hand Therapy*, and *Physical and Occupational Therapy in Geriatrics*, among others.

BNI

The recent launch of the **BNI** (British Nursing Index), jointly produced by the Royal College of Nursing and the University of Bournemouth, has provided the UK nursing and allied health profession with a new database in their area. Coverage starts from 1994 and approximately 220 journals are indexed. The thesaurus used is that previously produced by the Royal College of Nursing for its printed index, Nursing Bibliography. The therapy journals covered include: *British Journal of Occupational Therapy*, *British Journal of Therapy and Rehabilitation*, *Journal of Rehabilitation*, and *Physiotherapy*.

ASSIA

ASSIA (Applied Social Sciences Index and Abstracts) is strongest in its coverage of the social sciences. It has an advantage for a UK-based audience in its UK origins and coverage.

Access to general databases

Access to these databases is through a variety of media. Historically, print and online (via a telephone line) were the first to be made available, followed by CD-ROM (compact disc – read only memory) and the Internet. All six of the general databases are available in print. MEDLINE is available as Index Medicus, which is still taken by some of the larger university libraries. EMBASE is available as a series of subject specific publications and CINAHL comes as a bimonthly print publication and has been available since 1956. BNI is available in print form and is a cumulation of the former Nursing Bibliography and the Nursing and Midwifery Index. AMED is also available in print with topical sections available as separate publications. These topical sections are: Physiotherapy Index, Occupational Therapy Index, Rehabilitation Index, Palliative Care Index, and Podiatry Index. They are also available on floppy disk using a read only version of the *Idealist* software package. ASSIA is available as a printed index.

MEDLINE, EMBASE, CINAHL, AMED and ASSIA are available through online information providers (hosts). The two most important of these are **Datastar** and **Dialog**. To search these systems, you need a computer and a modem, but you will find that most healthcare libraries have access to online hosts and can help with searching the literature.

With the development of CD-ROM, most healthcare libraries have been able to offer many of these databases direct to their users. One of the first databases available on CD-ROM was MEDLINE, which is now produced by a number of CD-ROM vendors. The two major vendors, whose versions you are most likely to find in your local health library, are **OVID** or **SilverPlatter**, both of which offer easy searching interfaces and tools. CD-ROM has enabled most healthcare libraries to buy databases on subscription, eliminating the need for costly connection to online services. CD-ROM has led to the development of end-user searching where readers are encouraged to perform the search themselves, after training from the librarian. All of the databases are available on CD-ROM.

The advent of the Internet has led to some of the more common databases being made available for searching on the **World Wide Web** (www). For most of these a password is needed, and users are then billed by the organization making the database available. MEDLINE is being mounted free of charge by some vendors in an attempt to persuade users to use their sites and then access the other databases which have a fee attached. The quality of the versions of MEDLINE varies considerably and not all of them offer some of the more useful features. The E-lib project **OMNI** [http://omni.ac.uk] is attempting to list these sites and evaluate them against given quality criteria. BNI is already available on the Internet and it is anticipated that AMED will also be made accessible.

Using filters on general databases

If you are unable to identify relevant studies from specialist databases, such as the Cochrane Library outlined in the following section, you can, instead, filter the more important studies from the MEDLINE (McKibbon and Walker, 1993) or EMBASE (Cooke, 1996) databases. In other words, you can use the general databases as if they are in fact smaller databases of high-quality studies. For example, having completed a search on a particular treatment you can use the 'Limit' command in MEDLINE to restrict the results of your search to those studies with CLINICAL-TRIAL in the Publication-Type. This will give you a group of studies that meet the Cochrane Library's inclusion criteria. Similarly, if you retrieve too many articles from a MEDLINE subject search, you can use the 'Limit' command to restrict the results to those studies with REVIEW in the Publication-Type. Other useful restrictions include limiting your results set to the following Publication-Type: GUIDELINE, META-ANALYSIS or CONSENSUS-DEVELOPMENT-CONFERENCE. These so-called **quality filters** have also been devised for other types of study such as those dealing with diagnosis, aetiology or prognosis (Haynes et al, 1994).

Strategy B: specialist databases

Cochrane Library

Whereas the general databases include articles based purely on the merits of the journal in which they are published, a number of specialist databases attempt to focus instead on the quality of each individual article. So, for example, the **Cochrane Library** includes a register of over 150 000 controlled clinical trials from all subject areas, some of which predate MEDLINE's coverage (i.e. pre-1966). The criteria for inclusion of these articles are that each study will have both an intervention group and a control group. This will enable a comparison to be made between the effect of treatment in each group. A proportion of these will also include randomization as a means of deciding to which of two groups a patient or subject is allocated. The identification of these clinical trials is a long and painstaking process. This explains why coverage of some topics that have only recently begun to be featured, such as Therapy and Rehabilitation, is still quite poor. Nevertheless, this situation is changing with each successive edition of the Cochrane Library, so it is worth monitoring for the availability of appropriate studies.

As its name suggests, the Cochrane Library is not a single database, but rather a collection of databases available as a combined CD-ROM. The main database, the **Cochrane Database of Systematic Reviews**, currently contains the full text of over 200 systematic reviews produced by members of the Cochrane Collaboration. Each review has a standard format with sections that outline the methods, criteria for including studies, interpretation of findings and priorities for further research. This review database is also available on subscription via the Internet. The limited coverage of the review database is compensated for by the more comprehensive **Cochrane Controlled Trials Register**, referred to above. Here, however, you are presented with the raw materials of a series of bibliographic records rather than with a finished product. Because the register is compiled from a number of smaller registers, maintained by review groups, you will find that a number of references appear more than once. This can give the impression that there is more material on your topic than actually exists. A satisfactory compromise, between having the full version of a small number of reviews and brief details of thousands of controlled trials, comes with the **Database of Abstracts of Reviews of Effectiveness** where nearly 1000 reviews have been identified and brief structured abstracts provided by expert appraisers. Both these abstracts and the full Cochrane reviews use the Population–Intervention–Outcome anatomy referred to earlier. Finally, a number of support tools are contained in the database. These currently include a database of references on how to do reviews, the **Cochrane Handbook** on review methods and **Netting the Evidence: a ScHARR guide to evidence on the Internet**.

Best evidence

A recent addition to the high-quality evidence databases is the CD-ROM **Best Evidence**, produced by the American College of Physicians (distributed in the UK by BMJ Publishing who also market the Cochrane Library). Best Evidence contains the full text of both *Evidence Based Medicine* (1995 to date) and *ACP Journal Club* (1991 to date), two digest services that provide critically appraised commentaries on articles from major medical journals. Although not aimed primarily at a therapy audience, coverage of topics such as rehabilitation, orthopaedics and exercise testing make this a moderately useful source.

Specialist resources for therapists

The first stop for checking the literature must be your local healthcare library. This will be located either within your trust or within a local academic organization. The library will probably have access to MEDLINE, and increasingly the Cochrane Library, and can advise you on the best methods to access the literature. Many libraries will have CD-ROM facilities and are increasingly able to offer Internet access for users. There are, in addition, a number of major information centres that can be used by therapists.

The Chartered Society of Physiotherapy (CSP) Information Resource Centre

This is a national bibliographic information resource for physiotherapy. Its main role is to provide a support service for members who may have limited or no information resources locally. Services are available whether you write, telephone, visit, fax or e-mail the CSP. The largest collection in the CSP Information Resource Centre is its journal collection of over 140 journal titles. All important English-language physiotherapy journals are taken, along with other medical, nursing and allied health titles. Copies of many foreign-language physiotherapy journals from around the world are also housed in the Centre. A unique collection of journals, newsletters and other material produced by the various CSP clinical Interest and occupational groups is assembled for reference. A collection of members' dissertations and theses, which have been donated to the CSP, are located in the Centre. The CSP Physiotherapy Research Database is a register of current and completed physiotherapy research projects. Visitors to the Centre can carry out their own searches, having booked appointments. If you are unable to visit, then searches can be carried out on your behalf. Access is provided to over nine databases, including MEDLINE, CINAHL, AMED and the Cochrane Library. Current Awareness Bulletins and information papers are also produced. The Centre is open during CSP office hours, from 9.00 am to 5.00 pm, Monday to Friday. For further information and details of costs for services contact:

Senior Information Officer or Information Officer
The Chartered Society of Physiotherapy
14 Bedford Row
London WC1R 4ED
Tel: 0171 306 6604/5
Fax: 0171 306 6611

The College of Occupational Therapists Library and Information Service

This is available for members. It supplies information and advice to the profession and is accessible by telephone, written enquiry, fax, e-mail or personal visit. There are reference facilities, a collection of international occupational therapy journals, online searches and CD-ROM databases, including CINAHL and AMED, and the Internet and photocopies charged at cost. The Library produces Current Awareness Bulletins and factsheets. The Library will loan its collection of dissertations and theses. They can be contacted at:

Librarian
College of Occupational Therapists
106–114 Borough High Street
Southwark
London SE1 1LB
Tel: 0171 450 2316
Fax: 0171 450 2299

The British Library Reading Room

This is open to the public and has a large collection of clinical material and access to MEDLINE and EMBASE. Anyone can visit and use the collection, which is open from 9.30 am to 5.30 pm. It is located at:

9 Kean Street
Aldwych
London WC2B 4AT
Tel: 0171 412 7288

Internet sites

A number of specialist evidence-based healthcare centres have appeared around the UK and these can be useful sources of information and often have Internet sites. The **Centre for Evidence-Based Medicine** was the first of several centres. Its broad aims are to promote evidence-based healthcare and to provide support and resources to anyone who wants to make use of them [http://cebm.jr2.ox.ac.uk/]. Another member of the national network of centres is the **Centre for Evidence-Based Child Health**. The overall aim of the Centre is to increase the provision of effective and efficient child healthcare through an educational programme for health professionals. They offer introductory seminars, short courses, MSc modules, workshops for groups in the workplace and training secondments for healthcare professionals involved in child health. Their Web site is [http://www.ich.bpmf.ac.uk/ebm/ebm.htm].

A number of sites have set up pages of links to evidence-based resources. These are good starting points for listings and include:

- Cambridge University Public Health
  [http://fester.his.path.cam.ac.uk/phealth/phweb.html]
- Centre for Evidence-Based Medicine
  [http://cebm.jr2.ox.ac.uk/docs/otherebmgen.html]
- Health Promotion Research Internet Network
  [http://www.ki.se/phs/hprin/main.htm]
- McMaster University, Canada
  [http://hiru.hirunet.mcmaster.ca/ebm/]
- Netting the Evidence (ScHARR)
  [http://www.shef.ac.uk/~scharr/ir/netting.html]
- Oxford Clinical Information WWW Pages
  [http://users.ox.ac.uk/~clnguide/world.htm]
- South and West Health Care Libraries
  [http://www.epi.bris.ac.uk/rd/links/ebm.htm]

Journals

In the past, you have probably started your search for information with general journals such as *Physiotherapy*, *British Journal of Occupational Therapy*, *European Journal for Disorders of Communication*, *Archives in Physical Medicine and Rehabilitation*, etc. These journals are usually good at indicating issues of current concern, but do not necessarily focus on research that can be applied immediately to practice. In recognition of this, a number of specialist journals have appeared which aim to focus either on rigorous studies or on the methods for translating research findings into a clinical setting.

The *ACP Journal Club* was originally produced as a supplement to *Annals of Internal Medicine*. Its general purpose is to select, from the biomedical literature, those articles reporting studies and reviews that warrant immediate attention by physicians attempting to keep pace with important advances in internal medicine. These articles are summarized in value-added abstracts and commented on by clinical experts. The focus on internal medicine makes this journal of limited value to therapists. More useful is its sibling *Evidence Based Medicine*.

Evidence Based Medicine is published by BMJ Publications. Its purpose is to alert practitioners to important advances in internal medicine, general and family practice, surgery, psychiatry, paediatrics, and obstetrics and gynaecology, by selecting from the biomedical literature those original and review articles whose results are most likely to be both true and useful. These articles are summarized in value-added abstracts and commented on by clinical experts.

Following the successful launch of *Evidence Based Medicine* in 1995, a number of similar journals with specialist coverage are appearing with increasing frequency. First among these were *Evidence Based Nursing* and *Evidence Based Health Policy and Management*.

Bandolier is a journal produced monthly by the Oxford and Anglia NHS Region, in the UK. It contains bullet points of evidence-based medicine, hence its title. Access to *Bandolier* on the Internet is free of charge [http://www.jr2.ox.ac.uk:80/Bandolier].

The *Journal of Clinical Effectiveness* is a quarterly multidisciplinary journal, previously published as *Medical Audit News*, that addresses the linked concepts of methods of evidence-based healthcare, clinical effectiveness, clinical guidelines and clinical audit. It is published by Churchill Livingstone.

Both the *British Medical Journal* and the *Journal of the American Medical Association* (*JAMA*) have had a number of articles on evidence-based practice over the last few years and there are an increasing number in the therapy journals. The *JAMA* has actively publicized the writings of the Evidence-Based Medicine Working Group, who have created a set of guides, published in **The Users' Guide** series, which aim to assist practitioners to keep up to date in their clinical discipline and to find the best way to manage a particular clinical problem. The Users' Guides put much emphasis on integrative studies, including systematic overviews, practice guidelines, decision analysis, and economic analysis. They introduce strategies for efficiently searching and appraising the medical literature. Full text versions of some of the Guides are available on the Internet [http://hiru.hirunet.mcmaster.ca/ebm/userguid/default.htm].

Books

Books are beginning to appear on the subject of evidence-based healthcare. The main works include:

- *Evidence Based Medicine: A Practical Workbook for Clinical Problem Solving* (Dixon et al, 1997)
- *Evidence-based Healthcare: How to Make Health Policy and Management Decisions* (Gray, 1997)
- *Evidence-based Medicine: How to Practice and Teach EBM* (Sackett et al, 1997)
- *How to Read a Paper: The Basics of Evidence Based Medicine* (Greenhalght, 1997).

Finally, two recent resource guides act as a starting point for further information seeking: a publication from the British Library looks at the background to evidence-based medicine with an extensive bibliography and guide to sources and information centres (Grayson, 1997) while the *ScHARR Guide to Evidence Based Practice* (Booth, 1997) is also divided into a bibliography and a directory of resources.

Grey literature

Grey literature is loosely defined as being books or reports where there is no ISBN (International Standard Book Number) assigned. The term 'grey literature' includes material such as theses, conference proceedings and reports. Tracking this type of literature is difficult and the best place to start is usually the catalogue of your local healthcare library. The resource centres at the professional bodies are also a useful source. There are some specialist indexes in the field and these are: **Index of Conference Proceedings**, **Index to Theses**, and **British Reports, Translations and Theses**. The first two are published by the British Library and the third by Longman Cartermill. Some of the larger healthcare libraries will have copies of these publications.

However, there is one database of grey literature also provided by the British Library and that is called **SIGLE** (System for Information on Grey Literature in Europe). SIGLE provides access to records for reports and other grey literature from 1980 onwards in all subject areas produced in Europe. The database contains records from nine European countries, along with some of the R&D material produced by the European Communities. The majority of the material is in English. The file is updated monthly. Access to SIGLE is through BLAISE-WEB [http://blaiseweb.bl.uk] which is a fee-based service, or by CD-ROM marketed by SilverPlatter. The British Library also houses the National Reports Collection at Boston Spa and material is available for loan from that collection through your local healthcare library.

Current awareness

Keeping current and up to date with references is essential and a number of publications provide copies of title pages with a basic index. These are useful for searching within a limited time frame, but do not tend to produce cumulative indexes so are of no use for retrospective searching. The major ones are: **Current Contents: Social and Behavioural Sciences** and **Current Contents: Clinical Medicine**, produced by the Institute for Scientific Information (ISI) and taken by larger libraries. The British Library produces **Inside Science** and **Inside Social Sciences and Humanities**, which are similar but cover between them the 20 000 most used journals in the British Library. A further product, **Inside Healthcare**, is being planned which will be of more relevance to therapists. Both the ISI and British Library products are available electronically through CD-ROM or on the Internet.

Search strategies

The following three information-seeking scenarios will illustrate the process of finding the evidence. In each case two alternative means of seeking an answer to your question are examined, concluding with an evaluation of the effectiveness of each approach. They are presented as worked examples so that you can try them yourself.

MEDLINE versus EMBASE

MEDLINE and EMBASE are compared in Table 6.3 using the scenario presented at the beginning of this chapter:

A 35-year-old man is recovering from surgery after injuring his hand while cleaning the blades of his lawnmower ... He needs his hand to be fully functioning but is concerned that the time he may have to spend in rehabilitation would have a negative effect on his business ... You decide to search for evidence on the benefits of early as opposed to late intervention in rehabilitation following hand surgery.

AMED versus CINAHL

Starting with a more multiprofessional focus, AMED and CINAHL are compared in Table 6.4 using the following scenario:

You have been asked to treat an adolescent diagnosed with schizophrenia. You have access to AMED and CINAHL via your local library. Both AMED and CINAHL use a modified version of the MeSH headings.

Table 6.3 Scenario 1, MEDLINE versus EMBASE

MEDLINE (SilverPlatter version)	EMBASE (via the BIDS service)
#1. explode "HAND"/ injuries, surgery The explode function is a way of ensuring that not only will you retrieve documents indexed with the word 'HAND', but also those indexed more specifically under terms such as 'FINGERS' or 'THUMB'. From the list of 78 subheadings, most of which cannot be used with 'HAND', you selected **/injuries** and **/surgery** as the two most appropriate	**1. (early) @ (TI, AB, KWDS)** You start by focusing on the time factor, regarded as being so critical in our previous search
#2. explode "HAND-INJURIES"/ ALL SUBHEADINGS A number of parts of the anatomy also have their own assigned '-INJURIES' MeSH term. You decide not to restrict to any particular subheadings	**2. (late) @ (TI, AB, KWDS)** You decide that comparative studies that compare early versus late interventions may provide useful evidence of effectiveness
#3. #1 or #2 The two hand-related terms are combined into a single POPULATION set (#3) which will be used repeatedly in a number of different permutations	**3. (physiotherap*, management, physical therap*)** In light of your experience on MEDLINE you use the '*' truncation character. [NB. It just happens that the truncation character is the same on BIDS (EMBASE) as on SilverPlatter (MEDLINE)]. You are not using keywords (the equivalent to MeSH terms) specifically on this database, but the search option will pick them up if they happen to coincide with your search terms. This uses what are known as 'TREE STRUCTURES', whereby broad terms, *boughs*, such as 'HAND' include narrower terms, *branches*, such as 'THUMB'. Some structures include even narrower terms, *twigs*.
#4. explode "PHYSICAL-THERAPY"/ ALL SUBHEADINGS You now turn your attention to the INTERVENTION of interest, physiotherapy. Note that, as MEDLINE is an American database the preferred term is 'PHYSICAL-THERAPY'. The term is exploded so as to get all the more specific modalities that are included under this umbrella term	**4. hand, hands** The '*' character is not used for this step because there are too many potentially irrelevant variants, e.g. handle, handwashing, handicrafts, etc. It is best to think about the optimal position to place the truncation character
#5. #3 and #4 Here, for the first time the population and intervention groups are brought together to see where they overlap (i.e. any documents that are about hand injuries and physiotherapy)	**5. finger, fingers, thumb, thumbs** You don't have the explode feature here and therefore have to brainstorm other relevant subordinate terms. The comma ',' is equivalent to the MEDLINE expression 'or'

Table 6.3 continued Scenario 1, MEDLINE versus EMBASE

MEDLINE (SilverPlatter version)	*EMBASE (via the BIDS service)*
#6. #5 and (LA="ENGLISH") Up to now, despite the fact that MEDLINE is predominantly an English-language database, you have included non-English materials. This stage, which can be done easily by using the Limit command, eliminates non-English items	**6. 4,5** You create the hand-related set containing all the terms associated with the upper extremity
#7. #6 and EARLY Upon looking at the set of references you have retrieved in #6 above, you realize that you have not been able to introduce the critical factor of time. You therefore add in the free-text term 'EARLY' . Looking through this smaller set you see some potential references, many of which contain the index term 'TIME-FACTORS', which you thus decide to add to your search strategy	**7. 1&2&3&6** The ampersand '&' is the equivalent of the MEDLINE expression 'and'. Here you are looking for articles that mention physiotherapy, the hand and early and late. You decide to focus only on the 'early' articles
#8. #6 and "TIME-FACTORS" Notice that MEDLINE does not only index diseases, anatomy and treatments, but also other useful concepts that help in narrowing down a search. Usually, you will only identify these by reviewing your initial search results and seeing how relevant documents have been indexed	**8. 1&3&6** You find that there are not many relevant references and, because you are not using keywords exclusively, there is a high proportion of irrelevant documents (false positives, also known as 'false drops')
#9. EARLY MOBILIZATION You have come just as far as you can using the assigned MeSH terms. You will now have to depend on free-text words and phrases (i.e. those used by the authors in the titles and abstracts, not those words assigned by the indexers). One of your references uses the phrase 'EARLY MOBILIZATION' and therefore you decide to combine this concept with your hand injuries set (#3)	**9. EARLY MOBILI*** You can transfer the lesson from searching MEDLINE about the value of phrase searching and the need to use relevant truncation
#10. #9 and #3 At last you are approaching a suitable number of references. However, there are three flaws in your search strategy (#10). Can you identify them? 1. There are two different spellings of Mobilization/Mobilisation. As your search strategy stands you will find articles with one version in the titles or abstracts but will miss equally relevant articles with the other variant. A solution would be to use the wild card character '*' (i.e. Mobili*). This would also pick up 'Mobility', 'Mobilizing', etc.	**10. 6&9** A common issue for therapy searches is that therapeutic techniques may be applied to several anatomical regions. It is therefore particularly appropriate to combine the technique with the specific region of interest. As you review relevant articles you realize that many of the articles refer to tendon injuries. Not only does this have implications for the EMBASE search where you will want to type tendon, tendons, etc., but it might cause you to revisit the MEDLINE database! There is a predominance of surgery and orthopaedic journals but relevant

Table 6.3 continued Scenario 1, MEDLINE versus EMBASE

MEDLINE (SilverPlatter version)	EMBASE (via the BIDS service)
2. You are searching for the exact phrase 'Early Mobilization' but would miss related terms where the two words don't appear directly next to each other, e.g. 'Early Active Mobilization' or 'Early Controlled Mobilization'. You can avoid this either by using 'EARLY and MOBILIZATION IN TI, AB' (broad) or 'EARLY near MOBILIZATION' for the two words appearing in close proximity to each other.	journals include *Physiotherapy, Australian Journal of Physiotherapy, Physical Therapy* and *Physiotherapy - Theory and Practice*
3. You have forgotten to take into account synonyms such as 'EARLY MOTION'. There are as many permutations of these as there are of your first-chosen term.	

#11– #15 etceteras
#3 and (EARLY ACTIVE MOBILI*)
#3 and (EARLY CONTROLLED MOBILI*)
#3 and (EARLY ACTIVE MOTION)
#3 and (EARLY CONTROLLED MOTION)
#3 and (EARLY PHYSIOTHERAPY)
As well as looking at synonyms you will also need to make judgements about other related terms. For example, are you interested in continuous passive motion? If your search for evidence retrieves too many items (though not in this case) you may want to try limiting the results set to certain types of study, e.g. CLINICAL-TRIAL IN PT (publication type), RANDOMIZED-CONTROLLED-TRIAL IN PT, or REVIEW* IN PT

11–15 etceteras
6 & (EARLY ACTIVE MOBILI*)
6 & (EARLY CONTROLLED MOBILI*)
6 & (EARLY ACTIVE MOTION)
6 & (EARLY CONTROLLED MOTION)
6 & (EARLY PHYSIOTHERAPY)
On the EMBASE (BIDS) service result sets may be further refined by selecting the **Options** menu and limiting by language or publication type. You could also combine a search with the keyword 'RANDOMIZED CONTROLLED TRIAL' or with the keyword 'MAJOR CLINICAL STUDY'

Overall evaluation
You will have noticed from the above that a comprehensive search will usually require a mixture of MeSH and free-text terms. MeSH terms attempt to improve consistency, but free-text terms have a flexibility and precision which is not possible for MeSH terms

You will notice too that, because of MEDLINE's biomedical focus, the majority of references are from surgery or orthopaedic journals. The case study presented in Table 6.4 demonstrates the value of databases that are geared more to the therapy professions

Finally, MEDLINE is the longest established health database and this is reflected in the sophistication of the indexing language and functions such as the explode feature. MEDLINE is, therefore, the best starting point for a feel for the literature around a particular topic

Overall evaluation
EMBASE is not as easy to use as MEDLINE, particularly when accessed via the BIDS text-based interface. However, a World Wide Web version is now available which makes the stages of the search easier to follow

Although EMBASE does have an indexing terminology comparable to MEDLINE's MeSH terms, it is viewed, even by information professionals, as being unfriendly. Hence the high proportion of free-text expressions in this search. However, a review of relevant retrieved references will, once again, suggest the approved keywords as a starting point for further searching

Table 6.4 Scenario 2, AMED versus CINAHL

AMED (on DATASTAR)	CINAHL (on DATASTAR)
#1. Rehabilitation Rehabilitation is one of the main areas covered by AMED and so you know that there will be several articles on the subject	**#1. Schizophrenia with rehabilitation.de.** Unlike AMED, CINAHL treats rehabilitation as a subheading and so you can apply it immediately. CINAHL also has tree structures like MeSH and so you can search by tree number (F3.709.680.786)
#2. Schizophrenia Schizophrenia is a thesaurus term from AMED	**#2. #1 with allied with health.sb.** CINAHL allows you to select subject topics. This one selects allied health journals only but is limiting as CINAHL only indexes a limited number of allied health journals
#3. #1 and # 2 Combining the two terms will give you a smaller number of articles	**#3. #2 with adolescence.de.** Adolescence is a check-tag and so can be searched using the 'with' command
#4. #3 and (Young or adolescen*) If you find too many references you can use a free-text search to narrow down the number of articles to those dealing with young people or adolescents	**#4 ..limit/3 yr>90** Both AMED and CINAHL allow you to limit by date. Here you are looking for publications later than (>) 1990
Overall evaluation AMED is a small database compared to MEDLINE (90 000 references versus 500 000) AMED is composed of subject specific databases which are relevant to the therapy professions AMED uses a form of MeSH to control the indexing terms but is not indexed in depth	**Overall evaluation** CINAHL is a larger database than AMED but is primarily concerned with nursing literature CINAHL is indexed more closely to MeSH standards and uses check-tags and subheadings Rehabilitation is not one of the major topics covered by CINAHL

The Internet versus the Cochrane Library

With the increasing use of computers in the home and at work, the Internet is becoming widely accessible to both healthcare professionals and the public. Table 6.5 compares the Internet and the Cochrane Library using the following scenario:

A 17-year-old female was travelling home one Friday night with a group of young friends when the car that her boyfriend was driving careered off the road. Fortunately no-one was seriously injured but she presented to A&E with localized low back pain and was diagnosed with lumbar strain.

For some time you as senior physiotherapist for your unit have been considering whether the treatment you provide for low back pain is optimal or whether you might be offering an alternative. Stimulated by this young girl's situation, you decide that now is the time to conduct a brief investigation. You decide, firstly, to use your son's Internet connection to find some evidence and then, when you get into work, you will pop into the Library and perform a search on the Cochrane Library CD-ROM.

Table 6.5 Scenario 3, Internet versus Cochrane Library

World Wide Web (Internet)	Cochrane Library (compact disc)
1. URL: http://www.altavista.com/ The starting point for any search on the Internet, on any topic from architecture to zoology, is an all-purpose **search engine**. There are a number of search engines on the World Wide Web. Alta Vista is one of the largest and most powerful and it also allows phrase searching	**1. Select search button** Searching is at two levels, simple and advanced. You will usually find that the simple level is sufficient for your requirements
2. "low back pain" General purpose search engines cover so many documents that the more precise the query the more the likelihood of retrieving relevant documents. 'Low back pain' is better than 'back pain' because it is less likely to retrieve colloquial documents. Nevertheless, Alta Vista will still return over 1000 documents for this query, the first 10 of which will be displayed in short form. You will notice that although these are called 'documents' they are not documents in the true sense. Some are pages from academic research departments, others are teaching materials, and there will also be commercial services advertising chiropractic care, etc. For this reason you will probably be better catered for by a specialist medical search engine	**2. back AND pain** You enter your search statement as two words joined by the 'AND' relationship. This will look for all documents with both 'back' and 'pain' in them. Your results are displayed in the top window. For each of the six databases in the Cochrane Library you are presented with two figures, one for the number of results, *hits*, and the other for the total number of items in that database. You double-click on each line to get a list of hits and then double-click on an individual hit to view that document in the main window
3. URL: http://www.netmedicine.com/medfinder.htm This is a search engine that blends the variety of the Internet with the control of an indexing language. Instead of indexing the contents of documents automatically, each document is hand-selected for inclusion	**3. Cochrane Database of Systematic Reviews** This is rather unusual for a bibliographic database in that it contains the full text of systematic reviews (typically 10–20 pages). Results are divided into those that have been completed and those that are planned or in progress (protocols)
4. "BACK PAIN" **Medfinder Smart Search** has 74 sites with Back or Pain in them. One of the disadvantages of the multiplicity of search engines is that you can't know beforehand whether they combine words into a phrase or search for the words separately. Each document is given a brief title and is categorized, e.g. **Patient Information, Brief Review** or **In depth review/chapter.** If you enter a word or phrase which has common synonyms it will map your input to these other terms and then search for these terms as well as your original entry. Another specialist search engine is **Cliniweb**	**4. Database of Abstracts of Reviews of Effectiveness** This database contains structured abstracts that are halfway between an ordinary abstract and the full text of an article. Information on the review is placed against set subheadings and an evaluation of the usefulness of each article is made. A number of sources are listed as separate parts of the database including *ACP Journal Club* abstracts and reviews from Health Technology Assessment agencies

Table 6.5 continued Scenario 3, Internet versus Cochrane Library

World Wide Web (Internet)	*Cochrane Library (compact disc)*
5. URL: http://www.ohsu.edu/cliniweb Cliniweb maps your chosen term to its appropriate MeSH and then provides access to a list of resources grouped under the MeSH term	**5. The Cochrane Controlled Trials Register** By far the largest database in the Library, this contains references to clinical trials from sources such as MEDLINE. Where two or more groups have identified the same trial it will appear twice or more times on the database
6. "Low Back Pain" Cliniweb presents about 10 sites which have once again been evaluated and preselected. Typical amongst its coverage is the full text of a journal article, a critically appraised summary, two different versions of a US Government Agency for Health Care Policy and Research (AHCPR) guideline on low back pain and academic pages from Columbia University and the University of Iowa. Finally, we turn away from medical search engines to a structured resource list: the **Internet Database of Evidence Based Abstracts and Articles (IDEA)**	**6. The Cochrane Review Methodology Database** This will not usually have materials in support of a topic based search, such as back pain, above. It is more helpful when you want references on how to critically appraise articles or conduct a systematic review
7. URL: http://www.ohsu.edu/ bicc-informatics/ebm/ebm_topics.htm This is a list of documents indexed by MeSH term. All documents on this list show evidence of a literature search to identify high-quality evidence on the topic or include a critical appraisal of a single article. In this case you select the section K–M and browse down the list until you come to low back pain	**7. About the Cochrane Collaboration** This provides details of the groups or activities of the Cochrane Collaboration. For example you could check the activities of the Cochrane Musculoskeletal Injuries Group to see if it plans to produce reviews in your area
8. Low back pain You find at least four documents: the practice guideline from the AHCPR mentioned above; a critically appraised topic from the R&D journal *Bandolier*, a further practice guideline from the US Preventative Services Task Force, and a structured journal abstract from the *Journal of Family Practice Online*. However, success here is dependent on selecting the appropriate MeSH term. For example, had you looked on this list under the broader term 'back pain', you would have found nothing at all	**8. Other sources of information** The main content of this (at time of writing) is 'Netting the Evidence: a ScHARR Guide' which contains pointers to many of the sources listed in this chapter. It has been designed so that if the machine you are using is directly connected to the Internet you should be able to click on a link and proceed straight to the relevant document
Overall evaluation: The Internet offers all sorts of exciting prospects for delivering references or even full-text articles direct to your terminal. However, it is a sprawling chaotic,	**Overall evaluation:** All the materials on the Cochrane Library are higher quality and have been prefiltered. Along with MEDLINE, it should be one of your first ports of call

Table 6.5 continued Scenario 3, Internet versus Cochrane Library

World Wide Web (Internet)	Cochrane Library (compact disc)
almost anarchic, network of networks with no single responsibility for quality control. You have to make very rigorous checks on the source and origin of the information provided. If the last part of the Internet address (URL) of a source document has the tail **.edu** or **.gov** or **.nhs.uk** or **.ac.uk**, it is likely to prove of more value than a **.com** or a **.co.uk** extension General search engines are very powerful but yield materials of variable quality. If you search for materials by the scientific name of the condition or complaint you are more likely to match with the right type of sites. Conversely, the more colloquial the expression, the stranger your results will appear Specialist medical search engines are more likely to yield rigorous materials such as practice guidelines, critically appraised reviews, or single documents. Their limitation comes in the patchiness of their coverage, the delays caused by the appraisal process, and the variety of methods or standards used in their production	The materials included on the Cochrane Library are determined by the activities of the compilers. Unlike MEDLINE with its responsibility for completeness, some topics are covered well and others sketchily. The principal function of the database is to support the activities of the Cochrane Collaboration Unlike most of the Internet, the Cochrane materials attempt to evaluate or appraise their own usefulness or worth, hence the focus on structured abstracts

Cultivating lifelong information skills

The focus of this chapter, and the emphasis of evidence-based healthcare, is very much on the need to find information to answer a particular clinical question and to inform clinical decision-making. However, it is recognized that practitioners have two other major areas of information need that require evidence-based techniques and which are no less important (Williams et al, 1992). The first of these is the need to keep up-to-date in one's area of clinical expertise. For physicians to keep abreast of their speciality it has been estimated that they would have to read 133 articles a week (Davidoff et al, 1995). This is against a backdrop of their self-reported reading times of little more than 30 minutes a week (Sackett et al, 1996). The challenge facing therapists is little different in either magnitude or logistics for, as Barber (1995) writes, 'while the body of literature specific to many of the therapy and rehabilitation professions may be relatively small, the potential literature field is large and widely dispersed across related subject areas'. However a number of strategies might be suggested to keep this task within manageable proportions:

- Concentrate your reading time on critically appraised topics from digests and bulletins such as *Evidence Based Medicine, ACP Journal Club, Bandolier* and *Effective Health Care*

- Review each new edition of the Cochrane Library to identify new reviews, or newly identified randomized controlled trials in your areas of interest
- Cut down your reading of research articles to those with a rigorous study design, a form of comparison and where an attempt is made to discuss the applicability of the findings
- Focus your broader-based reading, not on opinionated editorials or correspondence, but on review articles where a systematic attempt has been made to cover the published literature
- Review evidence-based clinical guidelines such as those being developed by the Chartered Society of Physiotherapy's Clinical Interest Groups (Mead, 1996) and other professional organizations.

Similarly, the remaining area that also requires information skills is the more occasional need for a comprehensive search for all information on a particular topic. The time and effort taken for this particular approach should not be underestimated. Typically such a comprehensive search might cover up to seven different databases, all of which will usually have different search interfaces and search languages. Once again, however, the pursuit of this type of information can be made more evidence-based:

- Seek published reviews from the general databases or from the Cochrane Library database
- Check for the existence of compilations of the evidence by professional associations, academic bodies and governmental, or quasi-governmental organizations
- Seek to access not the original data but the interpreted syntheses of evidence, as incorporated in clinical guidelines.

In each of these circumstances, the secondary source (reviews, guidelines, etc.) may be used as a way of managing and accessing the references to primary sources. Of course, if there is no secondary source available then you can join the growing group of practitioners involved in producing evidence such as the volunteers of the Cochrane Collaboration or the researchers with funding from the NHS R&D programmes.

Keeping track of your references

Once you have performed your search and retrieved your references, you will find it helpful to maintain a file of those you have found useful. This will help you to locate them quickly and easily should you require them again in the future. The easiest way is to cut and paste the references onto index cards and then file them by author or according to topic. However, with computerization, a number of specialist software packages have been produced to enable you to download references from a database to your computer and then manipulate them for your word processor. All the following packages carry out the same sort of tasks, but they do vary in price. A networked version of one of these may be a good idea if a number of users want to access the same package. There are five main software packages available at this time, although others are appearing all the time.

Reference Manager

Reference Manager, by Research Information Systems, is perhaps the most well-known reference package. It delivers powerful features not found in any other software and is fast and flexible. You can enter references using the keyboard, or import from over 100 leading online, CD-ROM or diskette-based services. Reference Manager automatically creates lists of authors' and editors' names, keywords and journals. Research Information Systems offer a free demonstration copy from their Web site [http://www.pbsinc.com/rmprod.html]. Reference Manager includes more than 100 ready-to-use bibliographic formats and provides the capability to easily create any number of new styles. The software is available as Reference Manager for Windows, Reference Manager for DOS and Reference Manager for the Macintosh.

PAPYRUS

PAPYRUS is a product of Research Software Design, USA, and is similar in many ways to Reference Manager. You can type in your references or import them from existing computer sources. Working with your word processor, PAPYRUS will automatically assemble bibliographies formatted for publication. Dozens of predefined formats are provided for popular journals in many fields (biology, medicine, physics, chemistry, geology, etc.), plus several standard styles (e.g. Vancouver, Chicago and MLA). You may also modify any of these or create new formats from scratch. PAPYRUS Version 7.0 is currently available as a DOS program. This version also works under Windows 3.x, Windows 95, Windows NT, and OS/2, interacts with Windows word processors and supports copying and pasting from other applications. A free demonstration version is available at [http://www.rsd.com/~rsd/].

EndNote Plus

EndNote Plus 2 is available for Macintosh, Windows and DOS. EndNote Plus comes with more than 300 predefined bibliographic styles for the leading journals in a wide variety of disciplines, and you can easily create an unlimited number of your own styles. With **Endlink**, EndNote Plus's import module, you import these references into your EndNote Plus library without typing a word. More details are available at [http://www.niles.com/].

ProCite

ProCite is a powerful and full-featured reference management program for professional and personal use. You can also create your own electronic catalogue of publications, collections and research information. As with the other programs, you can build and maintain a local library of references from online, CD-ROM, and library systems and automatically generate properly formatted bibliographies of any type and in any style. ProCite comes with predefined bibliographic styles used by thousands of publications, including MLA, Nature, Science, and many more. You can use the **Biblio-Link II** utility program to import downloaded records retrieved from electronic database services. However, it should be noted that this is sold separately. You can network ProCite and it is currently available for use with Microsoft Windows, Apple Macintosh, and DOS. More details are available from [http://www.pbsinc.com/procite/procite.html].

Library Master

Library Master, the least well-known of these packages. It is a powerful, flexible and easy to use bibliographic and textual database manager. It automatically produces bibliographies, footnotes and citations for your paper, thesis or book. Unlike most database programs, Library Master does not require you to know how much information will go into a field when you create the database. All fields are of variable length and may contain up to 65 000 characters. The Library Master report generator is very flexible at formatting textual information. You can design a report that formats each type of record in different ways and handles exceptions such as empty fields and duplicate fields. Reports can be created in the file formats used by popular Windows and DOS word processors, including WordPerfect, Word and Ami Pro. Library Master imports from nearly 100 online information services, CD-ROMs, online library catalogues and other database programs. The Network Version gives inexpensive access by multiple users so that all users can edit and search the same database at the same time. A free demonstration version can be downloaded from the Internet at [http://www.gramcord.org/libinfo.htm].

Summary

This chapter should have prepared you for the first step in the evidence-gathering process, i.e. finding the evidence. Just as no two practitioners will have the exact same questions, no two questions will be similar either in their exact nature or in the sources that may provide answers to them. This has been demonstrated by the markedly different scenarios presented and by comparisons between matched pairs of information-seeking strategies. Help is at hand to assist you through this. First, use of the Problem–Intervention–Outcome–Comparison anatomy will assist you in arriving at a focused question, one that you or an information provider can adapt to the particular interface of a database, such as CINAHL. The memory aids that have been listed in the form of questions to ask yourself about your enquiry, will help you to decide on appropriate information sources, as will the published directories on coverage and access. Expertise in the use of both general and specialist resources is becoming increasingly available, together with the filters that allow you to extract those articles most likely to be clinically relevant. Software for managing your references and reprint collections completes the missing piece of the jigsaw. Meanwhile, health librarians all over the country are being trained under various initiatives to be more completely equipped to advise and support you. The evidence trail starts here!

Acknowledgements

Dave Roberts and Tony McCulloch of the British Library's Health Care Information Service are thanked for their invaluable help and expertise in preparing the AMED search example.

References

Antman, E. M., Lau, J., Kupelnick, B., et al. (1992). A comparison of results of meta-analyses of randomized controlled trials and recommendations of clinical experts. Treatments for myocardial infarction. *JAMA*, **268**, 240–8.

Barber, G. (1995). Searching the therapy and rehabilitation literature. *Br J Ther Rehabil*, **2**, 203–8.

Booth, A. (1996). In search of the evidence: informing effective practice. *J Clin Effect*, **1**, 25–9.

Booth, A. (1997). *ScHARR Guide to Evidence Based Practice.* School of Health and Related Research, University of Sheffield.

Bury, T., ed. (1996). *Introduction to Research.* Chartered Society of Physiotherapy.

Cooke, I. E. (1996). Finding the evidence. *Bailliere's Clin Obstet Gynaecol*, **10**, 551–67.

Dale, P., ed. (1997). *Guide to Libraries and Information Sources in Medicine and Health Care.* British Library.

Davidoff, F., Haynes, B., Sackett, D., et al. (1995). Evidence based medicine. A new journal to help doctors identify the information they need. *BMJ*, **310**, 1085–6.

Dixon, R., Munro, J. and Silcocks, P.B. (1997). *Evidence Based Medicine: A Practical Workbook for Clinical Problem Solving.* Butterworth-Heinemann.

Entwistle, V., Watt, I. S. and Herring, J. E. (1996). *Information about Health Care Effectiveness.* King's Fund.

Gray, J. A. M. (1997). *Evidence-based Healthcare: How to Make Health Policy and Management Decisions.* Churchill Livingstone.

Grayson, L. (1997). *Evidence Based Medicine.* British Library.

Greenhalgh, T. (1997). *How to Read a Paper: The Basics of Evidence Based Medicine.* BMJ Publishing Group.

Greer, A. L. (1987). The two cultures of biomedicine: can there be a consensus? *JAMA*, **258**, 2739–40.

Guyatt, G. H., Sackett, D. L. and Cook, D. J. (1994). Users' guides to the medical literature. II. How to use an article about therapy or prevention. B. What were the results and will they help me in caring for my patients? *JAMA*, **271**, 59–63.

Haynes, R. B., Wilczynski, N., McKibbon, K. A., et al. (1994). Developing optimal search strategies for detecting clinically sound studies in MEDLINE. *J Am Med Inf Assoc*, **1**, 447–58.

Lefebvre, C. (1994). The Cochrane Collaboration: the role of the UK Cochrane Centre in identifying the evidence. *Health Library Rev*, **11**, 235–42.

McKibbon, K. A. and Walker, C. J. (1993). Panning for applied clinical research gold. *Online*, **17**, 105–8.

Mead, J. (1996). Evidence based practice – how far have we come? *Physiotherapy*, **82**, 653–4.

Mulrow, C. D. (1994). Rationale for systematic reviews. *BMJ*, **309**, 597–9.

Reynard, K. W. and Reynard, J. M. E., eds. (1996). *ASLIB Directory of Information Sources in the United Kingdom*. ASLIB.

Richardson, W. S., Wilson, M. C., Nishikawa, J., et al. (1995). The well-built clinical question: a key to evidence-based decisions (editorial). *ACP J Club*, **123**: A12–A13.

Sackett, D. L., Rosenberg, W. M. C., Gray, J. A. M., et al. (1996). Evidence based medicine: what it is and what it isn't. *BMJ*, **312**, 71–2. (Also available on www http://cebm.jr2.ox.ac.uk/ebmisisnt.html).

Sackett, D. L., Richardson, W. S. & Rosenberg, W. M. C., et al. (1997). *Evidence-based Medicine: How to Practice and Teach EBM*. Churchill Livingstone.

Sheldon, T. and Chalmers, I. (1994). The UK Cochrane Centre and the NHS Centre for Reviews and Dissemination: respective roles within the Information Systems Strategy of the NHS R&D Programme, co-ordination and principles underlying collaboration. *Health Econ*, **3**, 201–3.

Smith, J. (1996). The National Centre for Clinical Audit: the first stage. *J Clin Effect*, **1**, 3–4.

Williams, R. M., Baker, L. M. and Marshall, J. G. (1992). *Information Searching in Health Care*. Slack.

7

Reading and critical appraisal of the literature

Tracy Bury and Christina Jerosch-Herold

Developing your reading habits

If you are to keep up-to-date and provide effective patient care based on sound evidence, it is important for you to develop and focus your reading habits. In order to practice effectively from day to day, anticipating what you might encounter, you will already need to be reading articles relevant to your speciality (Sackett et al, 1991). Regular systematic searching will help you in doing this. However, questions arising from practice that you are unable to answer, or are uncertain about, should also be the trigger for this approach, as outlined in the previous chapter. If you do not review new research regularly, you will not know when what you previously believed to be effective, is no longer the case!

Why might you turn to the research literature?

- To keep up-to-date: continuing professional development
- To answer specific questions arising from practice or services
- To pursue research
- To evaluate practice
- To prepare service specifications.

If you are reading regularly, you often rely on those sources of information which are easily accessible, for example, the journal that lands on your doorstep, which is part of your membership of a professional organization. Information that comes to you, rather than you having to go to it, is immediately more accessible. There are both advantages and disadvantages to this approach.

Advantages:

- It stimulates reading
- It is profession-specific
- It is easily accessible.

Disadvantages:

- You may miss important relevant articles
- You may change your practice inappropriately
- It may not provide a picture of the overall care and multiprofessional issues.

Chapter 6 has already highlighted the large volume of healthcare literature in existence, described the need to cultivate lifelong information skills and offered strategies for achieving this. In addition, Sackett and colleagues (1991) suggest the following tips:

- Invest some time in scanning journals to see which ones have the most high-quality articles of relevance to your particular field
- Discard from your reading list those journals with only limited or infrequent coverage of your topic (you may miss some relevant articles, but the likelihood is minimalized)
- Allocate dedicated reading time each week.

A word of advice: when you venture into the library, do not get sidetracked into reading a more interesting article which does not fit your purpose on that occasion. Losing an hour in a library is easy and you can still be no closer to answering the question that sent you there in the first place!

Why the emphasis on journal articles?

You will have gathered from what has already been said in this chapter that the focus is on research articles published in peer-reviewed journals, rather than textbooks. Why is this?

- The results of new research, which have been assessed by peer reviewers, usually appear first in the healthcare journals
- Journal articles provide an account of the study methods and results in enough detail to allow you, once your critical appraisal skills are developed, to assess the validity (truthfulness) of the findings and their applicability to practice (Sackett et al, 1991)
- Most healthcare literature is referenced fairly comprehensively in electronic form on one or more of the databases described in Chapter 6. This facilitates access to information
- The Internet is now making access to full text journal articles easier, although this is not widespread among therapy journals, as yet.

Whatever strategy has led you to particular articles, they will all need critically appraising for both quality and relevance to the question that initiated the search.

What is critical appraisal?

Critical appraisal is a systematic way of considering the truthfulness of a piece of research, the results and how relevant and applicable they are. One thing it is not is an attempt to pull a paper to pieces! In preparing to critically appraise a research paper it is important that you are open to new ideas and ready to challenge previously held beliefs. The assessment of the paper should start from the premise that there is probably no such thing as a perfect piece of research. This means that there will always be flaws in the papers that you read. What you need to consider is whether these flaws are important enough to make you question the conclusions arising from the research. The assessment should be balanced and constructive. Lessons can always be learnt and research improved upon.

Why critical appraisal?

Having obtained the literature, you are faced with the challenge of reading it. Being able to read a research paper, to assess its quality, is essential for lifelong learning and continuing professional development. It will help you to keep up-to-date and apply good research evidence in practice. Critical appraisal of the literature is an adjunct to clinical skills and designed to complement them.

Attendance at clinical courses is usually accompanied by a reading list, but little advice is offered about how to read the papers critically. However, this is beginning to change and should be encouraged.

When asked, many practitioners quote lack of time, confidence and familiarity with research methods and statistics as barriers to reading the research literature (Bohannon and LeVeau, 1986; Rubins, 1994). On reading a paper, you will probably feel confident reading the introduction and background sections. However, the same cannot be said for the middle section: the results and statistics. Tables and statistical abbreviations often appear as hieroglyphics and tend to be skipped. On reaching the discussion section, you may again feel more comfortable. However, a brief skip through a paper, missing several sections, can lead to:

- The authors' conclusions misleading you about the (in)effectiveness of an intervention, because they are not fully supported by the data
- Greater weight being given to those articles which reinforce previously held beliefs.

A critical appraisal of all sections of the research article helps to:

- Ensure a thorough assessment of all aspects of the research
- Encourage the implementation of effective interventions in practice
- Stimulate a greater appreciation of the contribution of research to the generation of knowledge
- Improve understanding of research methodology.

Learning and developing critical appraisal skills

Critical appraisal of research has to be learnt and practised like any other skill. There are a number of approaches that can be taken to acquire and develop such skills. Consideration also needs to be given to the necessary resources and support structures to facilitate this.

Professional education

The pre-qualifying education of occupational therapists and physiotherapists has made the transition from diploma to degree qualification within the last decade. Speech and language therapists made the transition earlier. One of the perceived benefits behind this change was that qualified practitioners would be better equipped to instigate research and to critically appraise and implement research findings within clinical practice. The type and level of journal readership among qualified physiotherapists, however, remains low, with only marginally higher use of journals among those with a degree (Turner and Whitfield, 1996).

A study of the information-accessing behaviour and use of research literature in clinical decision-making found that 90 per cent of interventions were based on what had been taught during initial training. Research literature ranked lowest, with review articles only marginally better, as a source of information for choosing interventions (Turner and Whitfield, 1997).

Such findings beg the question 'Has the transition of therapy education to degree level actually enhanced literature searching and critical appraisal skills among qualified practitioners?' While most undergraduate curricula include the teaching of research methods and the completion of a research project, it would seem that graduates are unable to base their practice on research evidence. Solomon and Stratford (1992) observed that second year students of a physiotherapy degree programme were unable to integrate their skills in critical appraisal with their clinical decision-making and treatment planning. They proposed that the fieldwork supervisor can play an evaluative role in assessing students' critical appraisal skills and provide opportunities for students to integrate research findings with patient care. This suggests that to successfully develop critical appraisal skills in undergraduates which will be maintained in their working practice, they need a supportive clinical environment which encourages this as part of routine practice. This in turn places a requirement on all practitioners to develop and maintain their critical appraisal skills, irrespective of when they trained.

Problem-based learning

The traditional educational approaches that focus on teacher-centred learning do not equip newly qualified practitioners for the challenges of the workplace, let alone to implement evidence-based practice. The use of lectures as a medium for teaching is inversely related to the development of effective clinical reasoning and self-directed learning (Barrows, 1986). **Problem-based learning** uses case studies to create a learning scenario that closely resembles the complexity, uncertainty and uniqueness of clinical practice (Schön, 1987).

The evaluation of different educational approaches is methodologically difficult, but some studies support problem-based learning. Bennett et al (1987) found that clinical clerks who were given instruction in critical appraisal skills using a problem-based approach demonstrated statistically and clinically significant better skills in critical appraisal than a control group.

This approach to teaching critical appraisal skills can be facilitated by using scenarios that relate directly to current clinical practice. These encourage you not just to develop skills in critical appraisal of research, but to relate this knowledge directly to patient care. For example, by using a structured format which includes questions about applicability, you are required to make informed decisions about how the research findings might be implemented into the management of individual patients, as the following scenario illustrates.

Clinical scenario

You are a senior therapist providing a traditional out-patient service to elderly clients in a community unit. You want to argue on the grounds of client-focused care that it is more appropriate to provide a home-based service.

You decide to see if there is any evidence of effective practice for this clinical problem and consult your librarian, who assists you with a search of the Cochrane Library database. You discover the following article:

Liang M. H., Partridge A. J., Gall V. and Taylor J. (1986). Evaluation of a rehabilitation component of home care for homebound elderly. *Am J Prev Med*, 1986; **2**(1): 30–4.

Having read the article, jot down your answers to the following questions:

1. Does a stepped up outreach rehabilitation programme improve function in older people with musculoskeletal disability?
2. Does this article provide you with evidence to support your case for a change in service delivery to a home-based programme?

Those involved in the development of any educational programme, whether at the pre-qualifying or post-qualifying level, should therefore consider the inclusion of clinical scenarios. Cooperation with practising practitioners will enable clinically relevant questions to be raised and translated into scenarios for the teaching of critical appraisal skills.

Example: the Critical Appraisal Skills Programme

One problem-based programme for teaching critical appraisal skills was instigated by the NHS Executive Anglia & Oxford Region Health Authority in 1994. The **Critical Appraisal Skills Programme** (CASP) was aimed at teaching the skills of critical appraisal of research literature to purchasers and providers alike (Gray, 1997). One perceived barrier to implementing evidence-based practice is that many health professionals may lack familiarity with research methods and statistics, which can impede clinical decision-making about groups of patients or individuals. CASP has run workshops to introduce professionals to the basic tenets of evidence-based practice and to develop their skills in critical appraisal. Workshops have focused on appraising a randomized controlled trial or a systematic review, using a structured format adapted from the **Users' Guides** for appraising literature (Guyatt et al, 1993, 1994; Oxman et al, 1993, 1994). Their aims are to:

- Encourage participants to plan and deliver further workshops at local level by providing 'training the trainer' days
- Cascade the skills through to all those involved in clinical decision-making
- Promote an evidence-based culture throughout the healthcare system.

Similar ventures have been developed in other health authorities. You can find out how to contact CASP by checking in Appendix 2 at the end of the book.

Lessons from the appraisal for clinical effectiveness (ACE) workshop

A programme that is aimed at a broad range of people with different remits within healthcare, such as the one delivered by CASP, can only fulfil broad aims. Teaching critical appraisal skills alone is not sufficient to ensure that therapists practise on the best evidence. They also need to acquire skills in finding the evidence as set out in the previous chapter.

The School of Occupational Therapy and Physiotherapy at the University of East Anglia (UEA), was commissioned by the NHS Executive Anglia & Oxford R&D Directorate to run a series of workshops for occupational therapists and physiotherapists, with the aim of developing evidence-based practice. The first two day workshop for senior managers included a half-day workshop on critical appraisal skills, run collaboratively between staff from CASP, faculty members from the School and staff from the Chartered Society of Physiotherapy (CSP), who already had experience of delivering such programmes. A 'finding the evidence' (CASP/few) workshop was run for the other half day by staff from the Health Care Libraries Unit, Oxford and local healthcare librarians. This involved practical hands-on searching using on-line databases, such as MEDLINE and CINAHL. On the second day the managers developed action plans required to develop an evaluative culture within their departments, which would provide the structures and support mechanisms for their clinical staff.

Having secured the enthusiasm and support of the senior therapy managers, a further two-day workshop was held for senior therapists. The critical appraisal skills workshop was adapted and delivered by faculty members from UEA and staff from the CSP (ACE workshop). It was attended by therapists from a wide range of specialities including the acute sector, mental health and community services. The teaching of critical appraisal skills to such an audience still warranted a generalist approach. A paper was therefore chosen to reflect a more general rather than specialist area of practice. This was followed by a workshop on finding the evidence (CASP/few). The second day concentrated on methods of implementing evidence-based practice through clinical audit, clinical guidelines and patient information.

The evaluation of the outcomes from this workshop is still underway and will be published in the future. However, the following points may serve as hints for those considering similar ventures:

- Adapting a CASP-style workshop to the needs of specific professional groups and providers of clinically specialist services allows a more focused approach. For example, the scenario and paper used for the critical appraisal skills part is more likely to be clinically relevant and allow participants to make informed decisions about questions of clinical applicability
- Opportunities are provided for networking among those working within the same clinical speciality, e.g. community mental health, and within a confined geographical area. Research development groups and journal clubs have been initiated by some
- The interdisciplinary nature of the workshop fosters collaboration between staff from the same unit, and may facilitate a shift towards more evidence-based practice at local level
- Opportunities exist for collaboration between practitioners and faculty staff in identifying gaps in the evidence. This may provide the impetus for research to be conducted in these areas which is also of high clinical relevance. Close links between faculty researchers and clinical specialists may lead to projects which will also attract funding.

Journal clubs

Journal clubs normally involve a group of people who meet regularly to review and discuss one or several journal articles about a specific topic. It has been suggested that critical appraisal skills improve with journal club participation (Linzer et al, 1988). Additionally, Burstein et al (1996) found that the use of a structured review instrument, such as a checklist of questions, further enhances the educational value of a journal club.

Journal clubs have been widely used by doctors (Linzer, 1987) and are becoming increasingly popular among many health professionals. Tibbles and Sandford (1994) see a journal club as a powerful educational tool used to introduce concepts of critical appraisal in the evaluation of research utilization. While students now learn these skills as part of their pre-qualifying education, others can acquire them through continuing professional development activities and participation in research journal clubs. Further benefits include shared decision-making about changes in clinical practice and consideration of the different perspectives that each participant brings to the discussion.

Format for a successful journal club

The formats for journal clubs can vary, and depend on the overall purpose of the meeting. Several authors (Brooks-Brunn, 1994; Tibbles and Sandford, 1994; Morton, 1996) recommend that meetings take place regularly on a monthly to quarterly basis. The leadership can be taken by a clinical specialist or someone experienced in critical appraisal skills; however, it should be rotated to enable each member to take a leading role. Where staff are relatively inexperienced or lack confidence in such an exercise, education programmes in critical appraisal should be provided. Articles should be distributed at least one week before the meeting to allow preparation, and preferably a tool should be used to structure the critique of the paper(s).

Kirchoff and Beck (1995) distinguish between different formats of journal clubs and their relative merits and shortcomings. Discussion of one article only per meeting allows these to be short in duration and to take place frequently. Such a journal club may be a good method for initiating the first meetings and allowing members to gain confidence. Its disadvantage is that the critique is limited to a single article and does not allow members to consider the breadth of evidence and discuss contradictory findings or replicated studies. It is therefore unlikely to lead to a change in practice. On the other hand, a journal club that considers several papers on a specific topic requires longer sessions and more preparation time. If preceded by a thorough literature search to select high-quality evidence, members can discuss conflicting findings and try to achieve consensus over a change of practice, based on current best evidence.

The membership of such a journal club need not be unidisciplinary. In fact, journal clubs held in a department are unlikely to meet the specific needs of practitioners working in a wide range of specialities. Discussing papers that are relevant to one's own clinical area is of greater value. Certain judgements about the trustworthiness of the research relate to the appropriateness of outcome measures, or whether the intervention used is practical and appropriate. Having some knowledge and experience in the field certainly helps in answering these questions. Articles should therefore focus on topics that are pertinent to the members' clinical area. Multidisciplinary membership of a journal club should also be considered, as decisions about a change in practice may require involvement of other members of the clinical team.

Barriers to a successful journal club

There are certain factors that may act as disincentives to those wanting to set up a journal club. If managers do not value research, they may not be willing to provide the resources such as time and library access. In the current healthcare climate, where managers have to be increasingly accountable for the services provided, this is less likely to be the case. In fact, a journal club can be a very effective method of surveying the research on a specific topic, especially if supported by a good-quality literature search provided by your local healthcare librarian, and if the load is shared among all the members of the journal club.

Another barrier may be an unwillingness to change practice. A journal club may find evidence that does not support a long-established and widely practised technique. Letting go of practices that have previously been favoured and valued can be difficult.

The most common problem, however, is the lack of high-quality evidence on therapy interventions that is accessible. Of the published studies, only a few will fulfil criteria for rigour and therefore be applicable to your own practice. However, a journal club may provide a forum where clinically important research questions can be identified and possibly instigated.

Research methods

This chapter is not about doing research. However, a range of commonly used research methods will be described briefly to assist you in understanding the terms encountered in research articles. For more detailed information you are referred to the further reading list at the end of this chapter.

Research methods are often described as either quantitative or qualitative. Quantitative approaches start from the perspective that there is a reality out there which can be studied and understood. Qualitative approaches take the view that reality is not a fixed entity and exists within a context which has many interpretations (Polit and Hungler, 1997). Table 7.1 provides a brief overview of some of the differences (Morse and Field, 1996; Polit and Hungler, 1997).

Qualitative investigation is often a prerequisite to good quantitative research, especially in areas that have had only limited investigation (Pope and Mays, 1995). This applies to many areas of practice involving

Table 7.1 Contrasts between quantitative and qualitative research approaches

Quantitative	Qualitative
Emphasis on testing theories/establishing relationships	Emphasis on developing theory
Setting is controlled, possibly artificial	Takes place in the individuals' natural setting
Control study variables as much as possible to reduce bias and increase precision	Emphasis on understanding human experience through analysis of beliefs, values, meanings, etc.
Data collection is primarily objective and measurable	Primarily rich subjective descriptive data collected
Narrow limited focus: exclusive	Generally broad focus: inclusive
Follows a logical series of predefined steps	Information collection and analysis can occur concurrently
Attempts to generalize beyond study participants	Less emphasis on generalizability

therapists. Quantitative research methods are necessary to investigate which treatment is more effective than another, for a defined group of patients. However, this invariably fails either to tell you whether the treatment is acceptable to patients, or to take account of their preferences. With developments in research methodologies, it is becoming more common for the approaches to be combined and the research to be staged to answer questions which do not simply focus on 'Does it work?', but also, for example, 'Is it acceptable?'.

As Mays and Pope (1995) stressed, 'All research is selective – there is no one way that a researcher can in any sense capture the literal truth of events. All research depends on collecting particular sorts of evidence through the prism of particular methods, each of which has its strengths and weaknesses'. Put in this context, you can see where descriptive studies, using qualitative approaches, will assist you in applying evidence of effectiveness in practice. Combining assessment of the literature from a range of methods will help you to take a more holistic approach to decision-making.

You will therefore come across a range of methodologies, all of which need to be critically appraised with equal rigour. Some of the most frequently encountered quantitative and qualitative methodologies are briefly outlined below.

Randomized controlled trial and controlled clinical trial

In a **randomized controlled trial** (RCT), participants are randomly allocated to one group or another, to receive or not to receive one or more interventions that are being compared. The results are assessed by comparing outcomes in the treatment and control groups (Mulrow and Oxman, 1997). A control group is important for providing a baseline against which the intervention group(s) can be compared. Explicit inclusion and exclusion criteria define who is eligible to enter the trial. Randomization is not always possible for practical or ethical reasons, and this can lead to the use of the **controlled clinical trial**. This still aims to compare one or more intervention groups with a control group.

Case-control study

In a **case-control study**, a group of people with a specific outcome or disease, such as stroke, are compared retrospectively with a control group who do not have the outcome or disease. The studies are designed to explore causal links between the outcome or disease and an attributable factor, such as a specific intervention or risk factor. This is achieved by comparing the frequency or level of the attribute in the cases and controls (Mulrow and Oxman, 1997).

Cohort or longitudinal study

A group of people, the **cohort**, is followed over time and outcomes are compared in subsets of the cohort who were exposed or not exposed to an intervention or other factor of interest (Mulrow and Oxman, 1997). For example, an intake of speech and language therapy students could be followed up over time to determine if specific pre-qualifying placements affect final choice of post-qualifying specialism.

Secondary research: systematic reviews and meta-analysis

The importance of systematic reviews was discussed in Chapter 1 in the discussion on what constitutes best evidence. A **systematic review** applies rigorous procedures to track down all previous studies relevant to a defined question, and to assess their quality. Data is extracted from the original research studies and analysed. A **meta-analysis** is a statistical technique used to analyse and summarize data from more than one study. It can be carried out if the individual studies are similar and of a high enough quality.

Ethnography

Ethnography provides a framework for studying meanings, patterns and experiences of a defined cultural group (Polit and Hungler, 1997). The aim of the researcher is to become an active participant, submerged in the cultural setting in order to learn from the group. The processes of questioning, information collection and interpretation take place concurrently. It can be used as a way of accessing the health beliefs of a cultural group, facilitating understanding of health and illness behaviour (Morse and Field, 1996; Polit and Hungler, 1997). It can be an important approach to understanding issues of acceptability, which in turn will impact on decisions concerning health service provision.

Phenomenology

Designed to promote human understanding, **phenomenological approaches** focus on the life experiences of individuals. The research aims to describe the experience and the individual's interpretation of it. The researcher is required to identify and put aside any preconceived opinions and beliefs about the phenomena being studied, so that they remain open to the interpretation of the experience by the individual. The research findings are not designed to be broadened to understand other groups (DePoy and Gitlin, 1994; Polit and Hungler, 1997).

Grounded theory

This approach aims to generate theories and explanations **grounded** in real world observations, based on the collection and analysis of qualitative data. The focus is the social and psychological stages that characterize an event or episode. Participants are therefore selected because of their knowledge of the particular topic or phenomenon being studied (DePoy and Gitlin, 1994; Polit and Hungler, 1997).

Statistics

Experience gained in teaching critical appraisal skills to physiotherapists and occupational therapists suggests that a basic understanding of the purpose of statistical tests and key terms helps therapists to gain confidence in assessing these sections of the paper. Therefore, this brief introduction to statistics is included. A further reading list is provided at the end of the chapter if you would like more detailed information.

The purpose of statistics

There are two basic reasons for using statistics (McCall, 1996):

1. They allow data to be described to provide general observations, referred to as **descriptive statistics**.
2. They allow conclusions or comparisons to be made from the population or sample, referred to as **inferential statistics**.

Descriptive statistics

One of the simplest descriptive statistics is the use of **percentages**. For example, 40 per cent of chronic asthma sufferers are female. You may want to know what value best summarizes the data. The common measures used are mean, median and mode.

The **mean** is the same thing as the average. It is calculated by adding up all the values of interest and dividing by the number of measurements. One problem of using the mean is when extreme values are included in the data, referred to as **outliers**. For example, the number of days between referral and assessment for a group of patients might be 6, 10, 7, 8, 7, 9, 8, 42. The mean for this group is 12. However, it does not fairly reflect the point around which most values lie. The **median** refers to the midpoint of a set of ordered data. If we order the days between referral and assessment recorded above (6, 7, 7, 8, 8, 9, 10, 42) we see that the median is 8. This number more fairly represents the central value. The **mode** is usually used with categories of data, such as social class, to describe the most frequent category.

These descriptions of the data do not tell you about the spread or variation within the data. The **range** indicates the difference between the highest and lowest scores. For example, subjects ranged in age from 42 to 86 years. While the range is 44 (86 – 42 = 44), this figure is rarely used as it is more informative to quote the lowest and highest score. The **standard deviation** (SD) summarizes the average distance of all scores from the mean of a set of data. The larger the standard deviation, the larger the spread of numbers observed. It helps to interpret the data gained from the participants in the study, not how it might relate to other patients.

Tables and graphs, such as pie charts, are another way of presenting data that allows you to get an overview of the results.

Inferential statistics

Research usually relies on a **sample**, selected from a **population,** in order to make it feasible to carry out. However, the idea is to make predictions about the population from whom the sample was selected. Ideally the sample should be selected at **random** so that each individual has an equal chance of being selected.

In order to use inferential statistics, a **null hypothesis** needs to be defined. This states that there is no difference between the interventions being compared in the study groups and that any observed relationship is due to the play of chance. The researcher's acceptance or rejection of the null hypothesis is therefore based on how probable it is that the observed differences are due to chance alone (Polit and Hungler, 1997).

The **level of significance** is used to indicate how confident the researchers can be that the results are not due to chance. This is commonly presented in papers as the P **value**. Convention usually means that the level of significance used is 0.05. This means that if you were to draw a number of samples from the population you would find similar results 95 times out of 100. Occasionally you will see 0.01 set as the level of significance. The P value can be presented as an actual result, such as $P = 0.23$, which in this case is not significant. Alternatively, the signs < (less than) or > (greater than) are used, e.g. $P < 0.05$ which is a significant result.

Statistical tests are then selected to test the null hypothesis. They are determined by a number of factors, such as the research question, the variables being compared, the sample size and the number of groups being compared (DePoy and Gitlin, 1994). These tests are used to calculate a value from which the level of significance can be determined, in order to accept or reject the null hypothesis. The researchers should have explained their choice of tests in the research paper.

Statistical versus clinical significance

Statistical significance does not equate to clinical significance. P values do not tell you about the size of the effect or the importance of the results to the clinical population (LeFort, 1993). However, to make an assessment of **clinical significance**, that is a clinically important change in practice, requires value judgements. This is likely to be informed by patients, carers and practitioners with experience of the area. It is these people who are in a position to decide if the clinical change makes a valuable contribution to an individual's quality of life, whether at a physical, emotional, social or psychological level. Measures such as confidence intervals, odds ratios and numbers needed to treat are more helpful in determining the effectiveness of interventions and their clinical significance.

Interpreting applicability and clinical benefit

Confidence intervals (CI) provide an estimate of whether the evidence is strong or weak. The CI is usually given as the 95% CI. It provides an upper and lower value within which you can be 95 per cent certain that the true result for any population lies. The narrower the CI, the more certain you can be about the true result (Fletcher et al, 1996). If you consider that the upper or lower limit of the confidence interval would still provide a clinically significant benefit, then the study has failed to exclude an important effect (Guyatt et al, 1994). Studies that have failed to demonstrate a beneficial effect should not be ruled out.

The **odds ratio** (OR) is used to provide a measure of benefit. An odds ratio of 1 means that there is no difference between the intervention and control groups. A value less than 1 means that there is less of the outcome of interest, whereas a value greater than 1 means that there is more of the outcome. If the outcome of interest is pain or mortality, then an effective treatment will have a value less than 1. If the outcome is function, then an effective treatment will have an odds ratio of greater than 1, because you want more of that outcome, as opposed to less.

Another relatively new measure of benefit which is gaining popularity is the **number needed to treat** (NNT). This is the number of patients who need to be treated to prevent one bad outcome (Mulrow and Oxman, 1997). For example, an NNT of 15 means that for every 15 people treated with the intervention, one person is prevented from having an adverse event. For an easy guide to calculating NNTs, see *Bandolier* number 36 (Moore et al, 1997).

Meta-analysis

An example of a meta-analysis showing effect sizes and confidence intervals, taken from a systematic review of relevance to therapists, is shown in Figure 7.1. This graph is taken from a paper by Aker et al (1996). It shows the effect of manual therapy on pain for individual studies and then as a combined result. The blob ● represents the result from the study and the line through it represents the confidence interval, the degree of uncertainty, also referred to as the *wobble factor*. Note how in some of the studies the confidence interval crosses the line of no difference, meaning that there is potentially no effect, or even a harmful effect. You can see that there was some disagreement between the studies and it was not until the results from the studies were combined to give an overall effect size that a clear beneficial effect was apparent.

The structure of research reports

Research articles are generally structured in a uniform way and consist of sections covering an introduction, methods, results, discussion and conclusions. Many start with a structured abstract which summarizes the key points from each section of the report. This is perhaps less common in the therapy literature and more suited to quantitative research.

From the **introduction section** you should be able to understand the rationale for the study. The summary of previous studies and

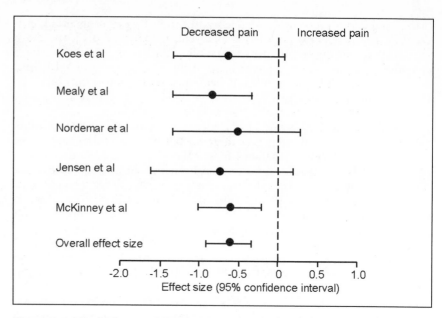

Figure 7.1 Effect of manual therapy on pain. (Reprinted from Aker P. D., et al. (1996). Conservative management of mechanical neck pain: systematic review and meta-analysis. *BMJ*, **313**, 1291–6, with permission.)

background knowledge sets the scene for this piece of research and defines its purpose. The **methods section** details how the study was carried out. Details of the processes of the study and the participants included or excluded should be set out. It is important that you have a clear picture of the study participants, for without it you will be unable to decide how useful this piece of research is in relation to your individual patients or population. This section should also detail the outcome measures that were used and the way in which they were applied. Reference should be made to the validity and reliability of the tools used. This section tells you a lot about the quality of the research.

The **results section** allows you to examine the findings of the study. This is usually presented in a combination of text, tables and graphs. Text is usually used to highlight some of the key results that the authors wish to draw your attention to. They should expand on and interpret the data contained in tables and graphs. There should be some descriptive data about the population, which are then followed by more detailed analyses. The importance placed on findings by the authors may not be the same as yours, so it is important to examine the data presented in tables and graphs to see if you agree. In qualitative studies, descriptive narrative is used alone, which is then condensed into themes and concepts. The results should fulfil the aims of the study; failure to do so raises concerns about the whole paper (Crombie, 1996).

The **discussion section** should allow you to examine the implications of this piece of work. Along with the description of the study participants, this will allow you to make a judgement about the relevance and applicability of this study to other individuals, populations or settings. The authors should offer a balanced perspective. Flaws in the study design should be acknowledged and their potential impact on the research discussed. Results should be interpreted with reference to previous studies, exploring differences and similarities. It is rare for research to come up with concrete conclusions and if presented as such they should be viewed with caution.

Checklists: providing a structured approach to critical appraisal

Purpose of checklists

The previous chapter has provided a structured and focused approach to tracking down relevant literature. If the same approach is applied to reading the literature, then you will use your limited time more effectively.

Checklists are designed to assist the reader in answering three key questions (Oxman et al, 1993):

1. Are the results of the study valid?
2. What are the results?
3. Will the results help me in caring for my patients?

Use of checklists

Checklists and tools for critical appraisal have been developed for studies concerning diagnostic tests (Jaenschke et al, 1995), prognosis (Laupacis et al, 1994), treatment and preventative interventions (Guyatt et al, 1993, 1994; Oxman et al, 1994) and clinical guidelines (Hayward et al, 1995; Wilson et al, 1995). In addition there are a number of books on the subject (Crombie, 1996; Sackett et al, 1997; Gray, 1997; Greenhalgh, 1997). Most checklists focus on quantitative research studies. However, there is a growing number that assess qualitative research (for example, see Forchuk and Roberts, 1993; Mays and Pope, 1995; Gray, 1997; Greenhalgh, 1997).

It is worth remembering that checklists are not going to tell you whether or not to act on the findings. Situations are rarely black or white, and decision-making relies on judgement in deciding on a course of action. As Oxman and colleagues (1993) said, 'Often results **may** be valid, **perhaps** demonstrate an important effect, and **might** improve patient care.' (emphasis added).

All of the resources and references concerning checklists mentioned above are of benefit to you in critically appraising the literature and have been used in defining the checklists which follow. Rather than having a number of checklists specific to each methodology, just two are presented. One is designed for primary research, irrespective of the method used, and the other for systematic reviews, because they need to be evaluated differently. They are divided into three sections of questions which cover:

- The validity (truthfulness) of the research
- What can be learnt, including the results
- The use of the research in understanding your own setting and decision-making.

Where quantitative and qualitative research approaches differ in their purpose and criteria for rigour this is indicated in the text. A summary of the checklist questions is provided in Appendix 1.

Checklist for primary research

Are the results of the study valid?

1. Did the research address a clearly focused issue?
Was there a clear aim to the research? Is there ample description of informants or participants and the context? In the case of clinical trials, strict entry criteria are used in order to increase the reliability of the study and this defines the population being studied. The outcomes being evaluated should be clearly stated, such as pain, mobility and anxiety. The other important element that should be clearly defined is the intervention. You should be left in no doubt as to what was being studied and in which environment.

2. Was the method appropriate to the question?
What was the study trying to do? For example, compare one treatment with another, or explore patients' beliefs about their illness? Considering the attributes of different methodologies, do you think the approach taken was the right one?

3. Was the sampling strategy appropriate and clearly explained?
Did the investigators sample the most relevant range of individuals and settings applicable to their question? Did they state their sampling strategy? Was there an adequate description of the participants?

For quantitative studies, the less control placed on the study design the more likely it is that other factors could have influenced the outcome. If appropriate, was random sampling used to minimize bias? Some samples are chosen for convenience and are therefore not random.

In qualitative studies, sampling takes place but participants are selected because they possess certain characteristics, have experience of the phenomenon being investigated or live in circumstances relevant to the investigation.

4. Were all of the participants who entered the study properly accounted for at its conclusion?
It is rare to find that all the patients who entered a research study are still involved at the end. Patients may withdraw or adhere poorly with the

treatment. However, they should still be included in the analyses. The greater the number who **drop out**, the more the validity of the study should be questioned.

In quantitative studies, excluding patients who have failed to adhere to treatment from the analysis potentially leaves behind those who may have been destined to have a better outcome, and this could lead to a biased comparison. Randomization is designed to reduce bias and therefore patients should be analysed in the group to which they were randomized, whether they dropped out or not. This is an **intention-to-treat** analysis (Guyatt et al, 1993).

Tip: The first four questions can be used as screening questions. If you answer no or can't tell to more than one, you need to consider if it is worth spending any more time on the article. However, you may need to revisit them later on. It is less appropriate to screen qualitative papers in this way because of the nature of the research.

5. Is the literature review appropriate?

Does it relate clearly to the purpose and focus of the research? Is it comprehensive and up-to-date? Does it draw on a range of sources? Weak reviews tend to be over-reliant on only one or two sources and to present only one view rather than presenting competing ideas (Finlay, 1997).

In qualitative research there are mixed views as to the timing of the literature review. Undertaking the review before commencing the study could potentially influence the researcher's perspective (Polit and Hungler, 1997). You will need to see if the researchers have justified their approach.

6. Were ethical issues considered?

Ethical considerations such as consent, confidentiality and the risks and benefits to participants should have been addressed (Forchuk and Roberts, 1993; Finlay, 1997).

7. Were measures taken to reduce bias?

(a) Were patients, healthcare professionals and study personnel blind to treatment?

In quantitative studies, an attempt should be made, where appropriate, to blind the practitioners involved in the study, so that they do not know if they are providing the actual intervention or control treatment, thereby not influencing the delivery of the intervention. Where possible, patients and carers should also be blind to the treatment, so that their behaviour and response are not influenced by knowledge of what they are receiving. This is difficult and unethical in many areas of rehabilitation. Those undertaking the observations and completing assessments of outcomes should not be influenced in their evaluation. To achieve this, they should also be blind to the allocation of patients. When participants know that they are part of a study they may alter their behaviour as a result. This is known as the **Hawthorne effect**.

(b) Did the authors make their role in the research clear?
You need to be clear what part the authors played in the research.

In qualitative studies, the researcher is required to interact with the participants, therefore a greater risk of bias exists. To overcome this, researchers can keep a reflective diary, designed to record how their beliefs and expectations may have affected the study or how they may have changed as a result of it. You should be clear about the researcher's role and motivation.

(c) Was the data assessed independently?
Did someone not involved with the intervention carry out the analysis of data? Was the analysis repeated by more than one researcher to ensure reliability?

8. Where a control group was used for comparison (quantitative studies only):
(a) Were the groups similar at the start of the study?
In clinical trials, if baseline comparisons are similar then it is likely that any difference at the end of the study is due to the intervention. Statistical tests should be used to examine if there are any significant differences between groups, often referred to as tests for **heterogeneity**. If groups in the study come from different populations, such as two general hospitals, they should still be compared for similarity. You may want to focus on other characteristics that could have affected the outcome, such as age, sex, social class or coexisting morbidity.

(b) Aside from the experimental intervention were the groups dealt with similarly?
The care given to experimental and control groups can differ in a number of ways besides the intervention. Differences in care other than that under scrutiny can weaken or distort the results (Guyatt et al, 1993). You must assess if the intervention was sufficiently standardized across participants. A feature often found in therapy and rehabilitation research is a comparison group where practitioners are advised to 'treat as normal'. This will result in different participants receiving different treatments. Problems arise if there are significant differences between practitioners or in treatment frequencies and duration (Vickers, 1995). The practitioner's competence can directly affect the results of the study. Ideally, details should therefore be given of their training and skills. The number of practitioners involved can also impact on the results. A positive outcome in a study involving only one practitioner may be due to the individual rather than the intervention. Generally, the greater the number of practitioners, the more applicable the results (Vickers, 1995).

9. Was there an adequate description of the method of data collection?
Data collection methods should be described and supported with a rationale. Consider how the data was collected. Were observations or measures taken at appropriate times?

In quantitative studies you need to check if valid and reliable tools and tests for assessing outcomes have been used, where appropriate. The outcome measures used should be referenced and their validity and reliability mentioned. If new tools, such as specifically designed questionnaires, are being used, the researchers should have carried out a pilot study to examine the validity, reliability and feasibility (ease of use) of the tool.

In qualitative studies, where the research involves an observer in the natural setting, there should have been sufficient time for the observer to become familiar with the setting, and for the participants to get used to having the observer present. How was the field work undertaken? Behaviours and events may vary depending on the time of day or other factors. You need to ask whether a wide range of activities was observed (Mays and Pope, 1995). Did data collection continue until no new information was being generated (Morse, 1991)?

10. Were the methods for data analysis appropriate, clearly described and justified?
Did they relate to the original research questions?

In quantitative studies, justification should be given for the statistical analysis used and the assumptions made about the data. Explanations of how extreme results were dealt with should be provided.

In qualitative studies it should be clear how the emergent themes and concepts were identified from the data. Did the investigator provide evidence of seeking out observations that might have contradicted or modified the analysis? How were negative or discrepant results taken into account? If there are some cases that appear to deviate from the researchers' explanations, they should have attempted to explain why (Mays and Pope, 1995). If appropriate, was the data fed back to participants for comment and verification?

What can be learnt from the paper?

11. What are the key findings?
Do the results address the research question? Are they likely to be clinically important?

In quantitative studies you should be able to identify the results for each of the outcome measures used, in all study groups. To assess the size of the treatment effect you need to consider the difference in outcomes between the groups. A measure of precision should also be provided in the form of a confidence interval or standard deviation. For both measures, the wider the range (variability), the higher the degree of uncertainty.

In qualitative research you need to check what the themes and concepts are that have emerged.

You will need to use your clinical judgement to decide if the findings would translate into benefits for patients in practice. If you discount them, there may still be useful information to be gained from the paper, such as the references cited (Crombie, 1996).

12. Is there sufficient detail to assess the credibility of the findings?
(a) Is there enough detail to assess the author's interpretation?
Is there sufficient original data presented systematically in the report to satisfy you of the author's interpretation of the results?

For qualitative studies, narrative descriptions should be presented systematically in the written account to satisfy you of the relation between the interpretation and the evidence. If quotations were used, were they numbered and sources given (Mays and Pope, 1995)? Is there sufficient original data presented in order to confirm how the themes and concepts emerged from the data? Have alternative explanations or theories for the results been explored and discounted?

(b) Are the findings reproducible and recognizable?
The method and data should be described sufficiently to allow another trained researcher to analyse the data in the same way and come to essentially the same conclusion. The account should also be recognizable to the participants.

Will the findings help you in making decisions?

Most research is intended to be relevant and applicable to wider populations than those included in the study population. Conclusions presented to support this must be closely examined. You need to consider whether the research will help you to have a better understanding of your local setting.

13. Can the findings be applied to your local population/individual patients/healthcare setting?
Will they help you to gain a greater insight into your setting and if so, how? Applicability is concerned with the transferability of the results to another setting or group. It refers to the degree of similarity between the two contexts. Responsibility for this lies with you, the reader, rather than the researcher (Krefting, 1991).

You need to consider the characteristics of the study participants to see if your patient(s) are similar to them. Where inclusion and exclusion criteria have been used, you need to consider if any of the exclusion criteria apply to your patients and how this might impact on the applicability of the findings.

The study may have taken place in a specific healthcare setting, such as an acute hospital. You need to consider if this limits the results being transferred to another setting, such as primary care or the community. As an individual, you may need to decide if you have the appropriate skills to deliver the intervention, and if not, what appropriate training is required.

14. Were all the clinically important outcomes considered?
This is really about quantitative studies. In order to assess if appropriate outcome measures have been used, you need a baseline level of

knowledge about the condition being studied. You need to ask whether they were appropriate for the condition and the intervention being studied. Were there any other outcomes that you would expect the researcher to have used? If you answer yes to this last question, you need to decide if this affects your decision or seek out further research to supplement the gaps.

15. Are the benefits worth the harms and costs?

Only now are studies beginning to include some form of risk–benefit analysis or economic valuation. This can make this question difficult to answer. The authors should have detailed any events leading to harm. Even if the paper does not include the relevant information, you need to try to answer this question. You should consider all possible factors that may deter a patient, practitioner or purchaser from using that intervention. Research concerning effectiveness alone is unlikely to provide you with all the information that you need to make an informed decision.

Checklist for review articles

Are the results of the review valid?

The first two questions are screening questions to assist you in using your limited reading time most appropriately. If you answer no or can't tell to one of them, you need to consider if it is worth continuing to a detailed appraisal.

1. Did the review address a clearly focused issue?

The same supporting information provided for the checklist for primary research applies here.

2. Did the authors look for the appropriate sort of papers?

The review will draw upon a number of studies in order to answer the research question. You need to consider if they are appropriate to the question and of a suitable study design.

3. Do you think important, relevant studies were included?

You need to check what databases have been searched to find studies. The previous chapter gives you some indication of those that would be appropriate. It is important that the search is not limited to one database. The authors should also have applied additional strategies, such as following up reference lists, contacting experts, searching for unpublished literature and non-English language studies. This is to reduce bias in the results. Publication tends to favour research that reports positive results, referred to as a **publication bias**. Also, researchers may tend to focus on writing up those studies which have supported their own ideas or have positive results.

4. Did the review's authors do enough to assess the quality of the included studies?

The authors should have critically appraised the individual studies against defined criteria. Two or three reviewers should be used, working independently and then comparing their assessments of the validity of the studies to be included.

5. If the results of the review have been combined, was it reasonable to do so?

In order to answer this question, the authors need to have provided you with sufficient information about the individual studies. From this you need to consider if the interventions being examined were similar enough and if the results were similar from study to study. Reasons for any variations in the results should be discussed. Are the results of the trials all or mostly pointing in the same direction? There is usually mention of statistical tests which have been used to examine the extent of any differences (heterogeneity) between studies.

What are the results?

6. What is the overall result of the review?

Specific outcome measures should have been identified. They will be limited by those used in the original studies. Results should be presented for all possible outcome measures. A measure of effectiveness mentioned earlier should be presented, such as NNTs or odds ratio.

7. How precise are the results?

The degree of uncertainty that surrounds the results should be presented with confidence intervals. The discussion under the primary research questions, concerning the key findings, applies here.

Will the findings help you in making decisions?

Questions to be addressed in answering this are the same as those presented for primary research.

Summary

Journal editors, in setting the style of research reports, often impose a word limit. This obviously limits how much information the researcher can include. That said, a well-written report should still provide enough detail for you to make a judgement about its quality and relevance. If you do pick some flaws in a relatively high-quality article, keep a balanced perspective. If they are real concerns that you need to resolve because the research is particularly relevant, then follow them up with the authors.

From this chapter you should be equipped to appraise a range of articles that you are likely to encounter in your practice, and to use your limited reading time more effectively. Critical appraisal skills are necessary for evidence-based healthcare and are vital if you are to be a competent practitioner, up-to-date with the latest research advancements, providing the best available care for your patients. They are also essential for managers, purchasers and policy-makers. You should feel more confident to use the literature to substantiate what you do, to develop new areas of practice or to abandon those areas which have been shown to be ineffective. Basically, critical appraisal skills enhance the decision-making process and make it more objective.

Acknowledgments

Barbara Richardson for permission to use the clinical scenario developed by herself and the authors for one of the critical appraisal skills workshops held at UEA. Workshops held by CASP helped to develop the ideas presented in this chapter and the authors are grateful for this experience. Barbara Richardson, Richard Stephenson and Britt van Royeen provided valuable comments on an early draft of this chapter.

Further reading

Statistics

Castle, W. M., and North, P. M. (1995). *Statistics in Small Doses*. Churchill Livingstone.
McCall, J. (1996). *Statistics: A Guide for Therapists*. Butterworth-Heinemann.
Rowntree, D. (1991). *Statistics Without Tears: A Primer for Non-mathematicians*. Penguin.

Research methodology: quantitative and qualitative

Bailey, D. M. (1997). *Research for the Health Professional. A Practical Guide*. Davis.
DePoy, E. and Gitlin, L. N. (1994). *Introduction to Research. Multiple Strategies for Health and Human Services*. Mosby.
Hicks, C. M. (1995). *Research for Physiotherapists. Project Design and Analysis*. Churchill Livingstone.
Morse, J. M. and Field, P. A. (1996). *Nursing Research. The Application of Qualitative Approaches*. Chapman & Hall.
Polgar, S. and Thomas, S. A. (1995). *Introduction to Research in the Health Sciences*. Churchill Livingstone.
Polit, D. F. and Hungler, B. P. (1997). *Essentials of Nursing Research. Methods, Appraisal and Utilization*. Lippincott.
Robson, C. (1993). *Real World Research*. Blackwell.

Epidemiology

Fletcher, R. H., Fletcher, S. W. and Wagner, E. H. (1996). *Clinical Epidemiology: The Essentials*. Williams & Wilkins.
Sackett, D. L., Haynes, R. B., Guyatt, G. H. and Tugwell, P. (1991). *Clinical Epidemiology. A Basic Science for Clinical Medicine*. Little, Brown.

References

Aker, P. D., Gross, A. R., Goldsmith, C. H., et al. (1996). Conservative management of mechanical neck pain: systematic review and meta-analysis. *BMJ*, **313**, 1291–6.

Barrows, H. S. (1986). A taxonomy of problem-based learning methods. *Med Educ*, **28**, 481–6.

Bennett, K. J., Sackett, D. L., Haynes, R. B., et al. (1987). A controlled trial of teaching critical appraisal of the clinical literature to medical students. *JAMA*, **257**(18), 2451–4.

Bohannon, R. W. and LeVeau, B. F. (1986). Clinicians' use of research findings. A review of the literature with implications for physical therapists. *Phys Ther*, **66**(1), 45–50.

Brooks-Brunn, J. (1994). Developing a unit-based journal club. *Nurs Management*, **25**(6), 80.

Burstein, J. L., Hollander, J. E. and Barlas, D. (1996). Enhancing the value of journal club: use of a structured review instrument. *Am J Emerg Med*, **14**(6), 561–3.

Crombie, I. K. (1996). *The Pocket Guide to Critical Appraisal*. BMJ Publishing Group.

DePoy, E. and Gitlin, L. N. (1994). *Introduction to Research. Multiple Strategies for Health and Human Services*. Mosby.

Finlay, L. (1997). Evaluating research articles. *Br J Occup Ther*, **60**(5), 205–8.

Fletcher, R. H., Fletcher, S. W. and Wagner, E. H. (1996). *Clinical Epidemiology: The Essentials*. Williams & Wilkins.

Forchuk, C. and Roberts, J. (1993). How to critique qualitative research articles. *Can J Nurs Res*, **25**(4), 47–56.

Gray, J. A. M. (1997). *Evidence-based Healthcare: How to Make Health Policy and Management Decisions*. Churchill Livingstone.

Greenhalgh, T. (1997). *How to Read a Paper: The Basics of Evidence Based Medicine*. BMJ Publishing Group.

Guyatt, G. H., Sackett, D. L., Cook, D. J., et al. (1993). Users' guide to the medical literature. II. How to use an article about therapy or prevention. A. Are the results of the study valid? *JAMA*, **270**(21), 2598–601.

Guyatt, G. H., Sackett, D. L., Cook, D. J., et al. (1994). Users' guide to the medical literature. II. How to use an article about therapy or prevention. B. What were the results and will they help me in caring for my patients? *JAMA*, **271**(1), 59–63.

Hayward, R. S. A., Wilson, M. C., Tunis, S. R., et al. (1995). Users' guide to the medical literature. VIII. How to use clinical practice guidelines. A. Are the recommendations valid? *JAMA*, **274**(7), 570–4.

Jaenschke, R., Guyatt, G., Shannon, H., et al. (1995). Basic statistics for clinicians. 3. Assessing the effects of treatment: measures of association. *Can Med Assoc J*, **152**, 351–7.

Kirchoff, K. T. and Beck, S. L. (1995). Using the journal club as a component of the research utilization process. *Heart Lung*, **24**(3), 246–50.

Krefting, L. (1991). Rigor in qualitative research: the assessment of trustworthiness. *J Occup Ther*, **45**(3), 214–22.

Laupacis, A., Wells, G., Richardson, S., et al. (1994). Users' guides to the medical literature. V. How to use an article about prognosis. *JAMA*, **272**(3), 234–7.

LeFort, S. M. (1993). The statistical versus clinical significance debate. *J Nurs Scholarship*, **25**(1), 57–62.

Linzer, M. (1987). The journal club and medical education: over one hundred years of unrecorded history. *Postgrad Med J*, **63**, 475–8.

Linzer, M., Brown, T., Frazier, L., et al. (1988). Impact of a medical journal on house-staff reading habits, knowledge and critical appraisal skills. *JAMA*, **260**, 2537–41.

Mays, N. and Pope, C. (1995). Rigour and qualitative research. *BMJ*, **311**, 109–12.

McCall, J. (1996). *Statistics. A Guide for Therapists*. Butterworth-Heinemann.

Moore, A., McQuay, H. and Gray, J. A. M. (eds) (1997). Calculating NNTs. *Bandolier*, **4**(36), 2.

Morse, J. (1991). Evaluating qualitative research. *Qualitative Health Res*, **1**(3), 283–6.

Morse, J. M. and Field, P. A. (1996). *Nursing Research. The Application of Qualitative Approaches.* Chapman & Hall.

Morton, S. A. (1996). Setting up a journal club. *Health Visitor*, **69**(11), 465–6.

Mulrow, C. D. and Oxman, A. D. (eds) (1997). Glossary. *Cochrane Collaboration Handbook* [updated September 1997]. In The Cochrane Library [database on disk and CDROM]. The Cochrane Collaboration, issue 4. Oxford: Update Software, 1997.

Oxman, A. D., Cook, D. J., Guyatt, G. H., et al. (1994). Users' guides to the medical literature. VI. How to use an overview. *JAMA*, **272**(17), 1367–71.

Oxman, A. D., Sackett, D. L., Guyatt, G. H., et al. (1993). Users' guides to the medical literature. I. How to get started. *JAMA*, **270**(17), 2093–5.

Polit, D. F. and Hungler, B. P. (1997). *Essentials of Nursing Research. Methods, Appraisal and Utilization.* Lippincott.

Pope, C. and Mays, N. (1995). Reaching the parts other methods cannot reach: an introduction to qualitative methods in health and health services research. *BMJ*, **311**, 42–5.

Rubins, H. B. (1994). From clinical trials to clinical practice: generalizing from participant to patient. *Controlled Clin Trials*, **15**, 7–10.

Sackett, D. L., Haynes, R. B., Guyatt, G. H., et al. (1991). *Clinical Epidemiology.* Little, Brown.

Sackett, D. L., Richardson, W. S., Rosenberg, W., et al. (1997). *Evidence-based Medicine. How to Practice and Teach EBM.* Churchill Livingstone.

Schön, D. A. (1987). *Educating the Reflective Practitioner.* Jossey-Bass.

Solomon, P. and Stratford, P. (1992). Promoting critical appraisal of research literature in undergraduate students. *J Phys Ther Educ*, **6**(1), 19–21.

Tibbles, L. and Sandford, R. (1994). The research journal club: a mechanism for research utilization. *Clin Nurse Specialist*, **8**(1), 23–6.

Turner, P. and Whitfield, T. W. A. (1997). Physiotherapists' use of evidence based practice: a cross-national study. *Physiother Res Int*, **2**(1), 17–29.

Turner, P. A. and Whitfield, T. W. A. (1996). A multivariate analysis of physiotherapy clinicians' journal readership. *Physiother Theory Practice*, **12**, 221–30.

Vickers, A. (1995). Critical appraisal: how to read a clinical research paper. *Compl Ther Med*, **3**, 158–66.

Wilson, M. C., Hayward, R. S. A., Tunis, S. R., et al. (1995). Users' guides to the medical literature. VIII. How to use clinical practice guidelines. B. What are the recommendations and will they help you in caring for your patients? *JAMA*, **274**(20), 1630–2.

8

Developing, disseminating and implementing clinical guidelines

Judy Mead

What are clinical guidelines?

The word **guideline** is defined in *The Concise Oxford Dictionary* (Sykes, 1982) as 'directing principle', and **clinical** as 'of or at the sick-bed'. So this suggests that a clinical guideline is something that provides guidance, in the form of principle(s), which can be applied to individual patients, at the point of the healthcare intervention. The National Health Service Executive (NHSE) definition similarly reflects the ethos of assisting decision making, primarily at a patient level. It states 'Clinical guidelines are systematically developed statements which assist clinicians and patients in making decisions about appropriate treatment for specific conditions' (Mann, 1996).

Guidelines have been written over many years. A number of clinical interest groups of the Chartered Society of Physiotherapy (CSP) have produced national guidelines for good practice, for example the Association of Chartered Physiotherapists in Oncology and Palliative Care (1993) and the Rheumatic Care Association of Chartered Physiotherapists (1994). The College of Occupational Therapists (1990), similarly, has developed guidelines, for example for documentation.

Such guidelines describe 'directing principles', but have an emphasis on the organizational framework within which a clinical intervention is given, rather than the intervention itself ['of or at the sick-bed', (Sykes, 1982)]. Where they do describe practice, the methodology for identifying recommendations is unclear. It is probable that most were based on informal consensus. However, the process of using panels of experts, or informal consensus, can easily be influenced by group dynamics, and recommendations may appear arbitrary (Huttin, 1997).

Clinical guidelines have a different emphasis. As indicated above, they provide recommendations for specific clinical interventions, which have been systematically developed (Mann, 1996). The key features of clinical guidelines are:

- The guideline recommendations are based on the best available evidence, i.e. a systematic and rigorous process has been undertaken to find, evaluate and synthesize evidence of effectiveness. Where research evidence is absent, of poor quality or provides conflicting evidence, the views of experts, patients' or professionals' experience, or consensus, will provide the best available evidence.
- Clinical guidelines deal with specific clinical interventions for specific patient populations, about which health professionals and patients need to make decisions.
- A systematic approach is taken to who is involved in the guideline development process. In all cases, patients' perspectives should be sought and used. It is rare for the interventions of a single professional group not to impact on other health professionals, or for other professionals not to have perspectives, skills or knowledge that can be used for the common good. For example, in developing a clinical guideline for physiotherapists using injection therapy (Association of Chartered Physiotherapists in Orthopaedic Medicine, 1999), general practitioners and rheumatologists had relevant contributions to make (Saunders, personal communication).

Such a differentiation between clinical guidelines about clinical interventions and organizational frameworks can be made clearly in relation to nationally developed documents. However, when national guidelines are being implemented locally, there will be a need to put the recommendations for clinical interventions in the context of local organizational systems, as will be shown in the dissemination and local implementation section of this chapter.

Why clinical guidelines?

A source of evidence of effectiveness for patients, professionals and policy-makers

In 1994, the Nuffield Institute for Health et al concluded 'the evidence ... strongly suggests that properly developed clinical guidelines can change practice and may lead to changes in patient outcome'. If a key feature of developing clinical guidelines is the synthesis and interpretation of the evidence for specific clinical interventions, this suggests that, if followed, they are an important component to achieve greater effectiveness for patients, reducing ineffective and inappropriate variations in practice. The ethics of delivering effective practice are discussed in Chapter 2.

Because of their reliance on a systematically developed evidence base, clinical guidelines are an important source of information about effectiveness. If clinical guidelines are developed rigorously, they will provide an important synthesis of the evidence for a particular set of circumstances, that is, the topic for the guideline and the population to which it applies. This is similar to the benefits of a systematic review. Indeed, most clinical guidelines use systematic reviews as key sources of research evidence, or develop a systematic review as part of the collection and synthesis of the available evidence.

So what is the difference between a systematic review and a clinical guideline? Is one more useful than the other? The added value of a clinical guideline is in its **interpretation** of the bottomline result of the review into recommendations for clinical practice, which take into account a range of perspectives, including those of patients.

For example, guideline development work pioneered in Buckinghamshire, as part of the Getting Research into Practice and Purchasing (GRiPP) project (Needham, 1994), was based on a review of research evidence (Coulter et al, 1993) which showed that there was no evidence of effectiveness for dilatation and curettage (D&C) carried out in women with dysfunctional uterine bleeding (heavy periods or menorrhagia). For women under the age of 40 years, in whom the risk of more serious disease was infinitesimal, the procedure was particularly questionable when weighed up against the risks of an invasive technique requiring a general anaesthetic. The project therefore aimed to reduce the number of D&Cs being carried out in these women, and to reduce variations in practice that had been identified across the county.

In order to change practice, it was necessary to involve a whole range of people with different interests, including general practitioners (GPs), consultant gynaecologists and public health doctors, as well as women sufferers and the media. GPs and consultant gynaecologists worked together to draw up a protocol (local guideline). Contract managers specified reduced levels of activity for D&C in women under the age of 40 in contracts, formalizing what had been agreed collaboratively between practitioners.

A key component was the development of information for women, to reduce the expectation that a D&C was the appropriate treatment. Women were involved in its development through the local consumer health information service, and through responding to calls for help in the local press. Reporting their experiences enhanced the relevance and appropriateness of the information, which was disseminated through leaflets and local media.

Clinical guidelines therefore present the evidence in the light of its application to clinical practice **and** patients' needs. They:

- Provide a format that can facilitate the implementation of research findings into practice
- Describe the evidence in the context of clinical applicability and a particular population
- Make clear recommendations, presented in an easily digestible format
- Provide a common information resource for patients and professionals,

which can balance the more usual asymmetry of information between them, facilitating partnership in decision-making.

Patients and professionals can make decisions based on the probability of good or bad outcomes (which should be described in the guidelines), taking account of their own experiences, preferences and risk assessments (Huttin, 1997). Clinical guidelines also provide an important information resource for patients to use as part of their decision-making process about their care, in order to give properly informed consent.

Patients should, wherever possible, be given a choice, and the use of clinical guidelines, even when set into contracts or service agreements, should not reduce this. The guidelines themselves should provide clear information about the implications for each choice, whether it be an increased risk or less likelihood of cure but increased quality of life. Guideline developers need to be mindful of the need to acknowledge potential differences in patient preferences, which should be accounted for in the guideline. The involvement of patients in the guideline development process has been described in Chapter 5.

Do clinical guidelines save money?

The assumption is sometimes made that clinical guidelines result in cost reductions. Guideline developers should certainly consider cost as well as clinical effectiveness. A cost–benefit analysis should be undertaken in order to provide information, on which guideline users can base decisions about using a particular clinical guideline in local practice. For example, if the cost is high and the evidence less than convincing (the evidence might be based on weak research methodology, results from studies may be conflicting or the degree of benefit may be marginal), a decision may be taken not to adopt the guideline locally. Guideline developers should present options where appropriate for the management of a particular set of clinical circumstances, to take account of both financial constrictions and patient preferences. These should weigh up the degree of clinical effectiveness of interventions, against the costs, patient acceptability, risks, harms and benefits.

The implementation of a particular clinical guideline may reduce costs directly or indirectly, for example fewer bed days if the number of D&Cs is reduced. Such savings could provide a cost reduction to the overall service, and would provide potential for an increase in other interventions of proven effectiveness. Equally, clinical guidelines may make recommendations for practice that will increase costs, for example the use of a newly developed, expensive drug.

Reducing inappropriate variation in practice

A high priority for clinical guideline development should be areas of clinical practice where there are wide variations in practice, particularly where some interventions are far more costly than others, or where there is evidence of some practices being more effective than others. While not technically a guideline, these principles can be illustrated by Effective Health Care Bulletin: *Total Hip Replacement* (Nuffield Institute for Health et al, 1996). This highlighted the wide variation in the quality and cost of hip prostheses being used in the UK. Research studies showed that two particular implants had the lowest long-term failure rate and in addition were among the cheapest. It was therefore recommended that these should be used more widely.

Clinical audit as a tool for implementing and evaluating evidence-based practice

Clinical audit is a key channel through which clinical guidelines can be implemented. The process includes the facilitation of change in personal practice behaviour and in organizational systems of care, as well as an assessment of the extent to which guidelines are used in practice. The use of clinical audit was highlighted in EL(93)115 (NHSE, 1993), which stated 'clinical audit will be an important means of assessing the extent to which guidelines are used successfully in practice'.

Clinical guidelines provide an opportunity to reinforce the importance of activity being measured against a set of predetermined explicit statements through clinical audit, as described in the next chapter. Once guidelines are in place, regular evaluation should take place to identify non-conformity, which might otherwise limit the opportunity of benefit for patients.

A tool for learning

As a source of evidence of effectiveness and an example of how evidence can be applied in practice, clinical guidelines provide an important resource for learning about evidence-based practice, at both pre-qualifying and post-qualifying levels.

Successful implementation of clinical guidelines locally requires the application of a number of steps in order to achieve an understanding of the content of the guideline and its applicability to their practice on the part of those who need to apply it. In going through such a learning process, a greater commitment to the application of the guideline, through a sense of involvement and ownership, is also likely. Factors could include:

- Consideration of the validity and applicability of the evidence presented in the guideline
- Exploration of the implications of the guideline's use in local practice
- Putting in place any changes in systems, or the skills or knowledge of those applying the systems, to ensure that the guideline can be applied in accordance with the recommendations
- Agreeing statements against which practice can be measured in order to determine the extent to which the guideline is being applied.

Placing these steps within the context of continuing professional development (CPD) will increase the potential for successful guideline implementation and should, therefore, be seen as steps within the implementation phase, described later in this chapter. Chapter 4 has also discussed the importance of CPD in getting research into practice.

Commissioning and purchasing services

When first introducing and promoting the value of clinical guidelines, the Chief Nursing Officer and the Deputy Chief Medical Officer wrote (NHSE, 1993).

> Clinical guidelines have been used by clinicians for many years. We now aim to work with the professions to identify and develop clinical guidelines which will be useful in informing discussions between purchasers and providers on the development of service specifications and contract negotiations. To be useful in this respect individual guidelines will need to satisfy a number of key criteria:
>
> - developed and endorsed by the relevant professional body;
> - based on good research evidence of clinical effectiveness;
> - practical and affordable;
> - where appropriate, multidisciplinary;
> - take account of patient choices and values.

However, the experience of the GRiPP project (Meara and Hicks, 1995), highlighted the limitations of using contracts as a way of ensuring more clinically effective practice. Imposition had negative connotations to providers of reducing practitioners' power or autonomy and cost cutting. The project concluded that developing trust, mutual understanding and partnerships with practitioners and others responsible for delivering services was more effective. Contracts were seen as a tool to give a signal about the importance of the evidence-based recommendations, but variables in particular situations made target-setting overly complex and counter-productive.

Clinical guidelines, if well developed, provide a useful resource for those making decisions about funding services as they comprise a clear description of the effectiveness of particular interventions for particular populations. The development of nationally relevant clinical guidelines, will provide the framework from which local quality standards can be agreed, for example between primary care groups and trusts, as part of their service agreements.

Legal implications of clinical guidelines

For professionals

- What **are** the legal implications of clinical guidelines?
- **Must** they be followed?
- Will guidelines lead to cookbook practice?
- Do clinical guidelines threaten clinical autonomy?

Remember the NHSE definition of a clinical guideline: '... statements which **assist** [emphasis added] clinicians and patients in making decisions about appropriate treatment ...' No guideline will apply to **every** patient in the population described in the guideline. There will always be exceptional circumstances in relation to some patients, for example, coexisting diseases, social factors or preferences. These will require individual practitioners to make judgements with individual patients about the appropriateness of that particular guideline for that particular patient. So clinical autonomy is alive and well, but so is responsibility. The CSP's (1995) *Rules of Professional Conduct* state clearly its underpinning philosophical principles: 'beneficence, autonomy and the professional's duty of care'. If a practitioner was to follow a guideline without considering its applicability to a particular patient, and it was to cause harm, this could be seen as a neglect of the duty of care, in other words, a **negligent act**.

Equally, compliance with guidelines is not a defence against liability if a practitioner's conduct in applying a guideline inappropriately was held to have been negligent. The test is, as with other medicolegal issues, whether a group of peers would have made the same judgement given the same set of circumstances. What has become known as the Bolam test is derived from a legal ruling in 1957 which stated 'the test is the standard of the ordinary skilled man exercising and professing to have that special skill'. The ruling also specified 'a doctor will not be guilty of negligence if he has acted in accordance with a practice accepted as proper by a responsible body of medical men skilled in that particular art' (Bolam v Friern Hospital Management Committee, 1957).

When applied appropriately, clinical guidelines should provide greater consistency of effective practice. They provide opportunities to reduce the incidence of those who do what they do because they have:

- Always done it that way
- A belief that an intervention works
- Read a case history and thought they would try it despite the lack of research evidence.

Opinion will become an increasingly unethical basis on which to found practice and will provide scant comfort in a legal setting, particularly where rigorously developed clinical guidelines are available.

Clinical guidelines will provide evidence that could potentially be used in court about expected practice. The appropriate use of clinical guidelines, compliance with which should be assessed through clinical audit, will therefore be a component of any professional's personal risk management, ensuring that the risk of harming patients or of being the subject of litigation is minimized. Copies of guidelines used must be retained, together with the dates when they were first used and ceased to be used, or were replaced by an updated version. They should be retained for at least as long as clinical records are required to be kept, i.e. eight years after the end of their use (CSP, 1993). In the event of litigation, the clinical guideline that was in use at any particular point in time can then be identified and can provide evidence of the appropriate bench-mark to practice at that time.

For guideline developers

Clinical guideline developers have responsibilities too. Hurwitz (1994) presents evidence that those who develop inadequate or flawed guidelines, or the application of whose guidelines lead to harm, may be held negligent. Third party organizations may be held liable if a clinical guideline is found to have caused a patient harm. This therefore adds emphasis to the need to develop guidelines rigorously and describe in detail how they were developed so that potential guideline users can assess the reliability of the recommendations.

Developing clinical guidelines

So, how do you go about developing a clinical guideline? What are the steps that need to be followed? The guideline development process described here is for rigorously developed, nationally relevant guidelines. The development of local guidelines is dealt with later in this chapter, in discussing local implementation, and in Chapter 9.

It is important to have an appreciation of the stages required to develop a national guideline so that you can critically appraise guidelines when they appear. It is also important so that you do not embark unwittingly on what is an enormous task!

Topic selection

Clinical guidelines are expensive to develop and require much time, effort, skill and commitment to implement successfully. It is therefore necessary to ensure that topics are chosen that are likely to give a good return for such investment. Topics need to be clearly focused, dealing with a discrete question, not a broad area of practice, for example stroke. The scope of the guideline needs to be clearly defined. Topics might be prioritized according to the following criteria (Mann, 1996):

- Where there is excessive morbidity, disability or mortality
- Where treatment offers good potential for reducing morbidity, disability or mortality
- Where there is a wide variation in practice around the country
- Where the services involved are resource-intensive: either high volume and low cost or low volume and high cost
- Where there are many boundary issues involved, cutting across primary, secondary and community care, and/or across different professional boundaries.

For therapists and patients, particular attention should be paid to the potential for:

- Health gain
- The guideline development process to provide new information about the most effective interventions, with priority given to areas where there is some research evidence
- Greater consistency of practice, rather than a lottery to determine which interventions patients receive depending on the practitioner or locality concerned
- Reducing risk
- More cost-effective and clinically effective practice
- Patient-centred, team approaches to effective practice.

Who should be involved in developing clinical guidelines?

Earlier in this chapter, some key features of clinical guidelines were described:

- Requiring a rigorous and systematic search for and evaluation (critical appraisal) of the research evidence
- The inclusion of expert or consensus opinion
- The involvement of a range of interested parties, including consumers
- The responsibility of the developers for ensuring that the recommendations are appropriate.

The responsibility of guideline developers to get it right from scientific, professional, ethical and consumer perspectives is therefore considerable. Strength in **academic** and **research skills** is important, as is **clinical expertise**, and also the **perspectives of consumers** and **other clinically relevant interested parties**. Those who have been involved in guideline development cite the importance of good project management and leadership skills and warn not to underestimate the value of efficient administrative support (Eccles, personal communication). Developing clinical guidelines is therefore a complex and lengthy business. A paper prepared for the Clinical Outcomes Group (NHSE, 1997) estimated the cost of developing a single clinical guideline to be around £50 000, not surprising when the numerous skill requirements, the wide range of interests and the lengthy process of synthesizing research evidence are all considered.

Once a topic has been identified, there is therefore a need to consider the involvement of any groups associated with that aspect of care. For example, the development of a clinical guideline for early treatment of the hand following injury or surgery (in preparation) involves specialist and non-specialist physiotherapists and occupational therapists, and hand surgeons. It might also have included patients who have experienced hand trauma or surgery, nurses and doctors from A&E departments, where patients with hand injuries first present, or nurses working on wards that deal with hand surgery. However, guideline development groups also need to be **manageable**, so the benefits of including all perspectives need to be balanced with achieving effective group dynamics. Those not involved directly can be targeted at the stage of consultation and piloting. Their feedback on the acceptability and achievability of the guideline will be crucial, particularly if they identify barriers to successful implementation. For example, a system may need to be developed for accessing speedy advice from experienced hand therapists for patients attending the A&E department.

One of the biggest challenges for clinical guidelines is to ensure their acceptability and applicability to consumers. This can only be achieved by the full participation of consumers in guideline development. Consumers will ensure not only that the search for and interpretation of the evidence has a consumer perspective, but also that the recommendations in the clinical guideline will be acceptable and applicable to them. They should include choices, where relevant, to take account of patient preferences. Arrangements for the involvement of consumers will need to be considered carefully to ensure their full and uninhibited contribution. Strategies may include extensive training for consumers, or the setting up of consumer-only groups that feed into the guideline development group, as described in Chapter 5.

Finding the evidence

Grimshaw and Russell (1993), in discussing factors which influence the validity of clinical guidelines, drew the following conclusions: '... guidelines developed without a literature review may be biased towards reinforcing current practice rather than promoting evidence-based practice'. In the same article, the authors discuss the role of consensus and expert opinion as a form of evidence. They acknowledge the importance of linking recommendations to the quality of the supporting evidence. In the absence of rigorously developed research evidence, recommendations can be based on other types of evidence. The **source of evidence**, and the mechanism for achieving it should be carefully described, so that the guideline user can estimate the reliability and relevance to their own practice, of each recommendation.

Guidance on finding the evidence can be found in Chapter 6. For a thorough and rigorous synthesis of the evidence, unpublished as well as published sources need to be explored. Expert sources and consensus opinion may need to be drawn on if the evidence is sparse or of poor quality. The following information should be provided:

- Databases used
- Key words used for searching databases
- Follow-up of references
- Conference abstracts
- Search for unpublished research
- International as well as national sources
- Non-English language as well as English
- How experts, if used, were selected
- How a consensus process, if used, was carried out.

Sufficient information should be included for the search for evidence to be repeated. Guideline users need to be confident that the process was a rigorous one, and that significant evidence was unlikely to be missed.

The process and validity of **consensus development** is poorly researched. However, a study of physicians working for the Harvard Community Plan in the USA demonstrated that when three groups of physicians were asked to develop a guideline for two similar clinical problems, the reproducibility of the consensus was poor (Huttin, 1997). This casts doubt on the validity of consensus development processes.

Appraising and rating the evidence

Chapter 7 deals in detail with the critical appraisal of research evidence. For clinical guideline developers, it is important to ensure that explicit and consistent criteria are used for the appraisal of the literature found. More than one person should carry out the appraisal of each paper independently, with the results being considered following this and an agreement reached on its quality. The research should be graded according to agreed criteria. The criteria recommended by the NHSE (Mann, 1996) are:

A Randomized controlled trials (RCTs)
B Other robust experimental or observational studies
C More limited evidence with the advice relying on expert opinion and having the endorsement of respected authorities.

Most published gradings of the evidence include systematic reviews as the gold standard evidence, which would be alongside RCTs (defined in the model above as grade A) as the most reliable form of evidence. While the use of a grading system makes it easier for guideline users to identify the reliability of the evidence presented, and its susceptibility to bias, a potential form of bias was highlighted by Newton and West (1997). The authors observed that while RCTs and systematic reviews continue to be the gold standard, biases could be introduced in clinical areas where these types of studies were inappropriate, for example rehabilitation and learning disability, discussed in Chapters 1 and 2. In these areas, no research evidence was likely to meet the perceived standard from which to draw the strongest recommendations for practice. However, the relevance of the research methodology to the question being asked is also important in assessing the evidence, as discussed in the previous chapter.

An evidence rating scale provides guideline readers with a clear indication of the strength of the evidence on which the guideline recommendations are based. Account of this can be taken when a patient is discussing choices and preferences about his or her care.

Making recommendations

There should be an explicit link between the clinical guideline recommendations and the supporting evidence. The strength of the evidence and grading of the recommendations helps with local adaptation, by indicating where there may be room for differing interpretations (Sudlow and Thomson, 1997).

An estimate of the costs, alongside the expected benefits, risks and patients' outcome preferences, should be discussed (Huttin, 1997).

Peer review and piloting the guideline

Once developed and at final draft stage, the guideline should be circulated for peer review and consultation. The target audience should include:

- Clinical experts in the field who have not been directly involved with the guideline development process
- Topic experts who will be able to check for gaps or inaccuracies in the evidence base and comment on the appropriateness of the recommendations in the light of the evidence
- Guideline methodologists, who will be able to comment on the validity of the guideline development process
- Potential guideline users, to comment on the guideline's acceptability, credibility and relevance to local practice.

Piloting of the guideline by a sample of users will elicit any problems with its practical application, together with its acceptability for patients and professionals alike. A judgement will then need to be made about possible problems arising from the pilot; whether the recommendations in the guideline itself need to be amended, without detracting from the evidence base. Problems may also need to be dealt with as part of the dissemination and implementation strategy, for example if barriers to implementation have been identified, such as skills or other resource gaps.

Presentation of the guideline

The presentation of clinical guidelines should facilitate their ease of use. Options include:

- Flowcharts and algorithms. These can identify key steps in the process and be used as a tool to highlight components that can be improved. They can be annotated to incorporate references to the literature and/or indications of the strength of evidence on which particular steps are based
- One- or two-page summaries, in the form of leaflets, pocket-sized laminated cards or posters, may be a useful way to make information more striking. Easy accessibility of these formats will promote their use, as well as have the potential to get over key points.

All guideline presentation should be reader-friendly. In addition, longer documents should be available to supplement brief summaries and algorithmic formats, which expand on the guideline development process, the evidence base and the rationale for the recommendations.

Attributes of clinical guidelines (adapted from Grimshaw and Russell, 1993)

- Do the guidelines lead to the health gains and costs predicted for them (**validity**)?
- Would another guideline development group, given the same evidence and using the same methodology, produce essentially the same recommendations (**reliability**)?
- Will guideline users, given the same circumstances, interpret and apply them in the same way (**reliability**)?
- Did all key affected groups participate in the guideline development process (**representative development**)?
- Is the patient population to which the guideline applies clear? Was the research evidence used in the guideline based on a similar population (**clinical applicability**)?
- Are patient preferences accounted for in the guideline? Are exceptions to the recommendations described? Is there enough information for you and your patient to make decisions about whether the guideline should be followed (**clinical flexibility**)?
- Is the language used in the guideline clear and unambiguous? Are terms clearly defined? Is it in a user-friendly format (**clarity**)?

- Does the guideline include a full description of the methodology used? Does it tell you who was involved and how the evidence base was established (**meticulous documentation**)?
- Is there a review date stated in the guideline? Is it clear who is responsible for the review (**scheduled review**)?

Responsibility for reviewing the guideline

Guideline developers have an ongoing responsibility to maintain and update the guideline, particularly in the light of new evidence of effectiveness. Other options for effective management may emerge, or new or reduced risk factors which may affect patient perceptions and choices. Each guideline should have a review date and, if necessary, arrangements made for funding to be made available for this to be undertaken.

Audit criteria

Guideline development should include the identification of explicit criteria against which the use of the guideline in practice can be measured through clinical audit. This is dealt with fully in the next chapter.

Desirable attributes of clinical guidelines

In 1993, Grimshaw and Russell identified a number of attributes of high-quality clinical guidelines, which summarize much of the discussion in this chapter. The attributes are to be aspired to by guideline developers and may be useful for potential users in determining whether a guideline has been developed appropriately, and therefore whether the basis of the recommendations is trustworthy.

Nationally or locally developed clinical guidelines?

The previous section about guideline development has highlighted the rigorous and extensive process that needs to take place in order to develop a reliable clinical guideline. It is therefore unsurprising to read 'development of guidelines requires considerable skill and resources perhaps beyond those available to most local or regional bodies' (Sudlow and Thomson, 1997). The authors go on to discuss, therefore, how the development of rigorous clinical guidelines is unlikely to happen in a widespread way locally. They observed that, at the time of their writing, the quality of national guidelines seemed to be greater than that of local or regional guidelines.

Equally, evidence suggests that guidelines developed by those who are to use them have the best chance of being used (Grimshaw and Russell, 1994). However, Sommers et al (1984) observed that guidelines developed locally by those who were going to use them may be seen as less credible than those developed with the involvement of locally respected practitioners (opinion leaders) or national experts.

So, while a rigorous approach to the guideline development process is more likely to be achievable at a national level, local ownership is essential to gain commitment to implementation locally. This suggests key processes need to take place locally, in order to achieve this.

Dissemination and local implementation of clinical guidelines

Dissemination

Developing clinical guidelines is a sterile, wasteful exercise unless they change behaviour to improve quality, effectiveness and benefit to patients. Effective dissemination is therefore crucial, to optimize the potential for making patients and professionals aware of the availability of particular guidelines, so that consideration can be given to implementation.

Dissemination of clinical guidelines is about providing information in an easy-to-use format to the right person at the right time either as a solution to an individual patient/practitioner problem, or in order to introduce a wider service improvement. The benefits of more than one strategy to get the message across has already been highlighted in Chapter 4.

The *Effective Health Care Bulletin, Implementing Clinical Practice Guidelines* (Nuffield Institute for Health, 1994), found that the mailing of information (mailshot) about clinical guidelines and publishing clinical guidelines in professional journals was unlikely to change professionals' behaviour, although it would raise awareness of the guideline. The Bulletin suggests that an additional, active educational initiative is needed to ensure use of the guideline in practice. For example, local meetings, in-service training or audit activities can all be used to focus on the use of a specific clinical guideline. 'Experts' (local opinion leaders) can provide a lead in achieving acceptance of the guideline. From a review of the literature concerning the likelihood of guidelines changing practice among doctors, Grimshaw and Russell (1994) concluded '... the more overtly educational the dissemination strategy, the greater the likelihood that the guidelines will be adopted within clinical practice'.

Members of the guideline development group can be encouraged to use their own professional networks to inform colleagues about the progress of the guideline as it is being developed, what it will mean for their practice, and why it is important, i.e. promoting the evidence base. The British Association of Hand Therapists plans to develop an educational pack for its members, including acetates for presentations. The Association will encourage its members to speak to local A&E departments, relevant wards, and non-specialist therapists about the implications for practice of the clinical guideline for the early treatment of the hand following injury or surgery (Birch, personal communication).

Which guidelines to implement locally?

There are three key factors to help you decide which guidelines to implement:

1. Is there a national guideline available?
2. Is it sufficiently rigorously developed to be confident of the recommendations? Does it have the endorsement of the NHSE, commissioners or professional bodies?

3. Is the implementation of the guideline likely to lead to significant health gain for the local population to whom the guideline applies?

Is there a national guideline available?

The availability of national guidelines is not always easy to determine as there is not, at the time of writing, a nationally recognized, comprehensive database of clinical guidelines of national relevance. Developing such a resource is fraught with difficulties, for example how to define 'national relevance' and how to decide whether or not a particular guideline appears in a database. Should there be some sort of quality control so that only well-developed guidelines are included? If so, what criteria would have universal acceptance and who would carry out the assessment?

Is the guideline sufficiently rigorously developed to be confident of the recommendations?

How do health professionals know if a nationally developed clinical guideline is suitable for use locally? The guideline may be endorsed (quality-checked) by the relevant professional body, or it may even be recommended by the NHSE. Any endorsement process should provide reassurance about the quality of the guideline development process.

However, the previous chapter on critical appraisal illustrated the importance of not believing everything that is written without a careful and systematic assessment of its trustworthiness and relevance (critical appraisal). Similarly, in order to decide whether or not to implement a clinical guideline developed by others, an assessment needs to be made of the extent to which the recommendations in the guideline can be believed, and therefore be used safely and appropriately locally. A number of models for the assessment of clinical guidelines have been published (Cluzeau et al, 1997; Hayward et al, 1995; Wilson et al, 1995). The key features to consider are precisely those that good guideline developers will have addressed, some of which are described in detail earlier:

- Is the guideline clearly focused, in terms of the population to whom and the clinical problem to which the guideline applies? Is my local population similar enough to the population for whom the guideline is intended to warrant local implementation?
- Was an appropriate range of people involved in the guideline process?
- Were all relevant sources of evidence sought, including consumer-led information?
- Was the evidence appropriately appraised?
- Do the recommendations in the guideline follow the evidence base as it was determined?
- Were there any vested interests? Was the development of the guideline funded by bodies that could predispose to certain biases?
- Was the make-up of the guideline group sufficiently broad and of sufficient experience that pressure from particular groups would have been balanced by other viewpoints?

Most users and assessors of guidelines will not have the resources to replicate the guideline development process, but there should be sufficient information in the guideline documentation to satisfy those interested, that an appropriate and rigorous process has been undertaken and that the results are therefore likely to be reliable. Such information is frequently presented as supplementary to the guideline recommendations, which are often published as easy-to-read, pocket-size leaflets. A fuller document should be made available to those who wish to look at the guideline development methodology and to examine the evidence base in more detail.

Is the implementation of the guideline likely to lead to significant health gain for the local population to whom the guideline applies?
The successful implementation of clinical guidelines requires considerable time and effort. The best strategies, already described in this chapter and in Chapter 4, are those that include educational initiatives, the involvement of a wide range of people, achieving local ownership, and feedback on performance, all highly time consuming. Yet without strong local commitment, it is unlikely that the guideline will be used. It is therefore important to ensure that topics for local guideline implementation are going to reap sufficient benefit to make the investment of time and energy worthwhile. For example:

- Is there some new evidence in the guideline that may not be currently considered best practice?
- Is the area one of high volume, high cost or high risk? These are likely to reap more gains, whether in health gain and/or resource allocation
- Is there currently variation in practice in the clinical area, through habit or preference, rather than considering the evidence of effectiveness?

Local implementation

While national clinical guidelines can provide a benchmark for local guidelines (Huttin, 1997), they will need to be tailored to local circumstances as part of an adaptation, or local guideline development, process. However, this does not mean that recommendations that are based on strong evidence can be tampered with.

Using a clinical guideline locally depends as much on organizational factors as on clinical validity and efficacy (Margolis, 1997). Systems and teamwork are at least as important to consider within the operationalization of the guideline as the specific recommendations for clinical intervention. Any changes in the process or system required to implement the guideline need to be identified, together with potential problems, barriers and causes that might hinder implementation. Are the barriers organizational, behavioural or financial? Systems may need to be reviewed to take account of such barriers if successful implementation is to be achieved.

Resistance to behavioural change is well described in Chapters 3 and 4. When implementing a national guideline, any of the following may provide barriers to change:

- Members of the local guideline development group may not be perceived as credible
- The reasons for change may not be clear or motivation may be poor
- Mistrust
- Perceived threat to clinical autonomy
- Too many other demands
- Perceived irrelevance to decision-making
- Medicolegal threat.

A useful summary of lessons about local implementation was identified by the GRiPP project, described in EL(94)74 (NHSE, 1994):

- Change should be managed locally
- Clarity about the expected benefits
- Thorough consultation and involvement
- Involve all interested parties
- Progress quicker with a **product champion**
- Constructive relationships between purchasers and providers
- Locally produced material essential, owned by those involved, but retaining the research basis of the national material

Table 8.1 Principles for adapting a national clinical guideline for local implementation

Feature	National focus	Local focus
The evidence	Synthesized Graded	Applied in clinical practice
Intervention	Defined	Defined and adapted within local systems, e.g. skill requirements resource implications skill mix referral systems educational needs
Recommendations	Broad statements	Local adaptation into measurable criteria
Presentation	Dissemination Documentation	Dissemination publicize market make available Implementation change management a defined group local information for patients and professionals
Follow-up	Review date	Evaluation in practice

- Contracting as a lever: to summarize agreements
- Time needed: no short cuts to thorough and detailed local work.

In developing a local guideline from a national guideline, explicit, measurable statements of performance and conformance targets should be agreed for monitoring purposes, as described in the following chapter. This will allow an assessment to be made about the performance that has or has not taken place.

Guidance on translating a national clinical guideline for local use is summarized in Table 8.1.

National initiatives may also, at times, be necessary to ensure that local implementation can take place. The *Clinical Guideline for the Management of Acute Low Back Pain* (Royal College of General Practitioners, 1996) identified manipulation as being effective during the first six weeks following onset of back pain. However, manipulation was not being taught routinely in qualifying programmes for physiotherapists. This raised national issues about the need for physiotherapists to be taught, at undergraduate level, those techniques for which there was strong evidence of effectiveness. There was some resistance, as manipulation was perceived to be a high-risk procedure and also not all educators involved with the teaching of musculoskeletal programmes had the required skill themselves. However, following an educative process about accepting evidence of effectiveness and dealing with the practical implications of developing these particular skills, all physiotherapists now qualifying should be equipped with manipulative skills (CSP, 1997).

The role of professional bodies in clinical guidelines

The NHSE's position is that 'the development, publication and maintenance of clinical guidelines remains the responsibility of the appropriate professional body, be it medical, nursing, dental or other' (Mann, 1996). The development of clinical guidelines contributes to the professional body's role of setting and maintaining standards. If this responsibility is to be accepted, professional bodies need to promote skills in guideline methodology. They also need to ensure that systems are in place for some form of quality control or endorsement of clinical guidelines. This is in order for the professional body to satisfy itself that any particular guideline that has been designed for national use has been appropriately developed and provides reliable information which will be of benefit to health professionals and patients alike.

Professional bodies also need to foster the effective dissemination and implementation of clinical guidelines. Sudlow and Thomson (1997) came to the conclusion that the resources and established communication networks of national bodies are likely to provide practitioners with easier access to guidelines. While professional bodies cannot directly ensure the local use of specific clinical guidelines, they can use their professional networks and other available channels to communicate expectations of local implementation.

Summary

Clinical guidelines provide a valuable synthesis of the available evidence of the effectiveness of interventions in particular circumstances. They have the added value of incorporating into the evidence base its clinical applicability and taking account of patient preferences and values. Well-developed clinical guidelines are an important information resource which provides patients and professionals with a level playing field on which to assess risks and benefits, from which decisions can be made.

Clinical guidelines are, however, expensive to develop, and the evidence that they will change practice or improve outcomes for patients remains scant. The potential for benefit, as statements based on the best available evidence, should add urgency to initiatives that focus on ensuring effective dissemination and implementation. Guideline development methodology is now well documented, if not always applied. Sound and straightforward methodologies are similarly needed to promote the effective **use** of guidelines.

Effective change management, local ownership and commitment to the evidence base are among key components for successful implementation. Each of these is concerned with learning, and can be set within the context of continuing professional development activities. Such an environment seems likely to have a good chance of achieving some success.

References

Association of Chartered Physiotherapists in Oncology and Palliative Care (1993). *Physiotherapy in Oncology and Palliative Care: Guidelines for Good Practice.* Association of Chartered Physiotherapists in Oncology and Palliative Care.

Association of Chartered Physiotherapists in Orthopaedic Medicine (1999). *Clinical Guideline for the Use of Injection Therapy by Physiotherapists.* Chartered Society of Physiotherapy.

Bolam v Friern Hospital Management Committee (1957). 2 All ER 118–128, 122

Chartered Society of Physiotherapy (1993). *Standards of Physiotherapy Practice.* Chartered Society of Physiotherapy.

Chartered Society of Physiotherapy (1995). *Rules of Professional Conduct.* Chartered Society of Physiotherapy.

Chartered Society of Physiotherapy (1997). PA40. *Guidance for the Safe Teaching of Manipulation to Undergraduates.* Chartered Society of Physiotherapy.

Cluzeau, F, Littlejohns, P., Grimshaw, J., et al. (1997). *Appraisal Instrument for Clinical Guidelines.* St George's Hospital Medical School.

College of Occupational Therapists (1990). *Guidelines for Documentation.* College of Occupational Therapists.

Coulter, A., Klassen, A., MacKenzie, I. Z. et al. (1993). Diagnostic dilatation and curettage: is it used appropriately? *BMJ*, **306**, 236–9.

Grimshaw, J. and Russell, I. (1993). Achieving health gain through clinical guidelines I: Developing scientifically valid guidelines. *Qual Health Care*, **2**, 243–8.

Grimshaw, J. M. and Russell, I. T. (1994) Achieving health gain through clinical guidelines. II: Ensuring guidelines change medical practice. *Qual Health Care*, **3**, 45–52.

Hayward, R. S. A., Wilson, M. C., Tunis, S. R., et al. (1995). Users' guide to the medical literature. VIII. How to use clinical practice guidelines. A. Are the recommendations valid? *JAMA*, **274**(7), 570–4.

Hurwitz, B. (1994) Clinical guidelines: proliferation and medicolegal significance. *Qual Health Care*, **3**, 37–44.

Huttin, C. (1997). The use of clinical guidelines to improve medical practice: Main issues in the United States. *Int J Qual Health Care*, **9**, (3), 207–14.

Mann, T. (1996). *Clinical Guidelines: Using Clinical Guidelines to Improve Patient care within the NHS*. Department of Health.

Margolis, C. Z. (1997). Methodology matters: VII. Clinical practice guidelines: methodological considerations. *Int J Qual Health Care*, **9**(4), 303–6.

Meara, J. and Hicks, N. (1995). Bringing it together: the GRiPP experience. In *Clinical Effectiveness from Guidelines to Cost-Effective Practice* (M. Deigham and S. Hitch, eds) pp. 123–6, Department of Health.

Needham, G. (1994). A GRiPPing yarn – getting research into practice: a case study. *Health Libraries Review*, **11**, 269–77.

Newton, J. and West, E. (1997). Clinical guidelines: an ambitious national strategy (editorial). *BMJ*, **315**, 324.

NHS Executive (1993). EL(93)115. *Improving Clinical Effectiveness*. Department of Health.

NHS Executive (1994). EL(94)74. *Improving the Effectiveness of the NHS*. Department of Health.

NHS Executive (1997). *Clinical Outcomes Group CG3/97: National clinical guidelines project bids 1997/98*. Department of Health.

Nuffield Institute for Health, University of Leeds and NHS Centre for Review and Dissemination, University of York (1996). Effective Health Care Bulletin: *Total Hip Replacement*, **2**(7), Churchill Livingstone.

Nuffield Institute for Health (1994). *Effective Health Care. Implementing Clinical Guidelines*. Bulletin no. 8. University of Leeds.

Rheumatic Care Association of Chartered Physiotherapists (1994). *Guidelines of Good Practice for the Management of People with Rheumatic Diseases*. Rheumatic Care Association of Chartered Physiotherapists.

Royal College of General Practitioners (1996). *Clinical Guideline for the Management of Acute Low Back Pain*. Royal College of General Practitioners.

Sommers, L. S., Sholtz, R., Shepherd, R. M., et al. (1984). Physician Involvement in Quality Assurance. *Med Care*, **22**, 1115–38.

Sudlow, M. and Thomson, R. (1997). Clinical guidelines: quantity without quality (editorial). *Qual Health Care*, **6**, 60–1.

Sykes, J. B. (ed). (1982). *The Concise Oxford Dictionary*. Oxford University Press.

Wilson, M. C., Hayward, R. S. A., Tunis, S. R., et al. (1995). Users' guides to the medical literature. VIII. How to use clinical practice guidelines. B. What are the recommendations and will they help you in caring for your patients? *JAMA*, **274**(20), 1630–2.

9
Implementing evidence through clinical audit

Yvette Buttery

Introduction

Clinical audit is an important mechanism for facilitating the use of evidence in practice. The primary objectives of this chapter are to provide you with a step-by-step approach to clinical audit. It will offer enough knowledge for you to be able to establish audit as an effective tool with which to promote evidence-based practice in your workplace. First, the scene will be set by providing you with a brief history of clinical audit. Some general discussion, in particular about what is termed here as evidence-based clinical audit, is followed by a guide through the different stages of the clinical audit cycle.

History of clinical audit

Practitioners have always undertaken activities to assess and improve the quality of health services. In the therapy professions, for example, professional standard-setting has been advocated for some years (Chartered Society of Physiotherapy, 1993; College of Occupational Therapists, 1990; Royal College of Speech and Language Therapists, 1996). This is also the case in nursing (Royal College of Nursing, 1980, 1981), while in medicine, activities have, for many years, included mortality and morbidity review (Royal College of Physicians, 1990). Various confidential enquiries, such as the confidential enquiries into perioperative deaths (Buck et al, 1987) and maternal deaths (Department of Health, 1991a) have also been in place. To a large extent though, until the National Health Service (NHS) reforms were introduced in 1989, activities to assess and improve the quality of health services in the UK were undertaken largely on a voluntary basis.

With the implementation of the NHS reforms, the informality of quality assessment and improvement activities changed markedly (Department of Health, 1989). With the support of some of the medical Royal Colleges (Royal College of Physicians, 1990; Royal College of Surgeons, 1990), the Department of Health directed all providers in the NHS in England to develop audit programmes which would involve all doctors in the critical analysis of their practice. A year later, this was extended to include all members of other clinical professions (Department of Health, 1991b).

What is clinical audit?

The term **clinical audit** means different things to different people. Indeed, a wide range of activities are undertaken in the name of clinical audit. This chapter focuses on the use of clinical audit to implement evidence into practice. This can be categorized as:

- Activities that aim to achieve the widespread adoption of best clinical practice or management by agreeing, then implementing, explicit statements of best practice, thereby achieving changes in practice.

Other categories that some would consider audit, which are not considered here, include:

- Activities that aim to identify real or potential quality problems. This includes monitoring activities such as regular patient satisfaction surveys, Patient's Charter monitoring and outcomes monitoring. Such monitoring activities can highlight areas that need improvement which might subsequently become the focus of specific projects aimed at solving these quality problems.
- Surveys of current practice. This sort of activity is often undertaken with a view to informing practitioners about the nature of their practice in order to assist them in developing guidelines, protocols or standards of care or management. However, the danger of this is that there is no way of knowing whether current practice is best practice, unless the evidence is considered, as described in this chapter.
- Assessments of outcomes before and after changes in practice have been made. The usual reason for undertaking this kind of assessment is the desire to find out what impact changes in practice have had in terms of outcomes for patients, referred to in Chapter 4.

With clinical audit being used in different ways, many definitions exist. However, the definition set out in the working papers which accompanied *Working for Patients* (Department of Health, 1989), subsequently adapted (NHS Management Executive, 1994), has now gained a common currency:

... the systematic critical analysis of the quality of clinical care, including the procedures used for diagnosis, treatment and care, the associated use of resources and the resulting outcome and quality of life for the patient.

This definition focuses on the **assessment of quality**, but does not mention explicitly **quality improvement**. Clinical audit is commonly visualized as a cyclical process combining quality assessment and quality improvement (Walshe and Coles, 1993), producing continuous improvements in quality (Fowkes, 1982) as illustrated in Figure 9.1. Indeed, the NHS Executive's (NHSE) most recent definition reflects the cyclical nature of clinical audit and focuses on both quality assessment and improvement:

> Clinical audit is a clinically led initiative which seeks to improve the quality and outcome of patient care through structured peer review whereby clinicians examine their practices and results against agreed standards and modify practice where indicated. (NHSE, 1996a)

As Figure 9.1 shows, the clinical audit cycle comprises a number of stages:

- Agreement of guidelines, protocols or standards
- Implementation of guidelines, protocols or standards
- Assessment of compliance with guidelines, protocols or standards (involves data collection and analysis)
- Agreement of changes (if required)
- Implementation of agreed changes.

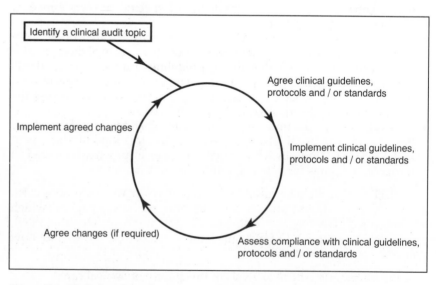

Figure 9.1 Clinical audit cycle.

Since clinical audit aims to generate continuous improvement, it is usually necessary to repeat the cycle a number of times, usually referred to as re-audit.

Each of these stages will be addressed more fully in later sections. However, it is important to clarify two things: first, the difference between clinical audit as described here and audit and feedback as presented in Chapter 4; and, second, what is meant by the terms guidelines, protocols and standards.

Clinical audit compared with audit and feedback

Oxman and colleagues (1995) define **audit and feedback** as any summary of clinical performance of healthcare provided over a specified period of time, with or without recommendations for clinical action (see Chapter 4). They consider two types of feedback: passive and active. They categorize passive feedback as the unsolicited provision of information with no stated requirement for action, and active feedback as that which engages clinicians in the process.

If you compare the model of clinical audit shown in Figure 9.1 with Oxman and colleagues' definition of audit and feedback, you will see that the latter is much narrower. It includes neither the agreement and implementation of guidelines, protocols or standards, nor the agreement and implementation of changes. Moreover, it makes no explicit reference to the repetition of the audit cycle. Rather, it focuses on the measurement of practice performance, with or without recommendations for action. Data collection and analysis therefore form a more significant part of the activity than they do in the clinical audit cycle presented above. According to this cycle, while data collection and analysis are important, the other stages of the clinical audit cycle are just as important. Indeed, without them, you will not be undertaking **good** clinical audit (Buttery et al, 1995).

Guidelines, protocols and standards

Guidelines, protocols and standards all provide explicit statements of best clinical practice or, in other words, explicit statements of expected practice performance. The terms **guidelines**, **protocols** and **standards**, together with other similar terms, are often used interchangeably, which can be confusing. The important point, however, is that clinical audit, as described here, is not possible in the absence of some form of explicit statements of best clinical practice.

The NHSE (1996b) defines a clinical guideline as 'systematically developed statements which assist clinicians and patients in making decisions about appropriate treatment for specific conditions'. However, the definition is usually associated with a particular type of clinical guideline: a **national clinical guideline**, which has been developed and implemented in a particular way, described in Chapter 8. In practice, there are many definitions relating to clinical guidelines, and also to protocols and standards. This is partly because different professions have different definitions. In view of this, definitions will not be offered here. Rather, it is important that when you get involved in clinical audit activity, you clarify with all involved what everyone means by the various terms and come to an agreement about working definitions. By doing this, you will avoid not only confusion, but also potential alienation of colleagues in other professional groups, by accepting that their definitions are just as valid as your own.

In general terms though, it is the level of detail these various forms of explicit statements of best practice contain that provides the main difference between them. While guidelines tend to contain broad statements about what and how patient care should be provided, protocols and standards usually contain more specific statements.

As you will see from Figure 9.1, the agreement of explicit statements of best practice in the form of locally applicable guidelines, protocols or standards comprises the first stage of the clinical audit cycle. Nationally relevant clinical guidelines will almost never be developed locally as part of the clinical audit cycle because of the resources required to develop and implement them (see Chapter 8). However, the **adaptation** of a national clinical guideline to a local context, that is, the formulation of a local clinical guideline based on the recommendations contained within a national clinical guideline, is commonly undertaken in a local setting as part of the clinical audit cycle.

What is evidence-based clinical audit?

Since 1996, the NHSE has not treated clinical audit as a stand-alone initiative but, rather, has promoted it as a component of a much more wide-ranging one: clinical effectiveness (NHSE, 1996c). This aims to enhance the degree of clinical effectiveness of services to patients by getting evidence into practice (see chapter 2). So, what has changed about clinical audit?

The principles of clinical audit have, in fact, not changed. Indeed, clinical audit's overall aim of quality improvement remains unaltered, as do the stages of the audit cycle. The change is one of focus rather than substance, such that greater attention is now paid to ensuring that the practice being evaluated through clinical audit is based on the best available evidence. Chapters 1 and 2 described evidence as being derived from three main sources: research; clinical expertise; and patients' preferences and experiences (NHSE, 1996c). Ideally, best practice should be determined by research. However, the reality is that the research base for many areas of practice is rather sparse. In the absence of research-based evidence, you will need to rely on evidence derived from clinical expertise. Importantly, though, whether there is any research based evidence to determine what is best practice or whether this has to be based on clinical expertise, evidence derived from patients' values and preferences must always be combined to provide a holistic picture (see Chapter 5).

In the past, it was not uncommon for a group of professionals or even an individual to develop explicit statements of best practice (whether called a guideline, protocol or standard) based largely on their own personal beliefs and experiences about what constitutes best practice (see Chapter 1). That is not to say that these did not provide an adequate description of best practice. The important point is that the use of evidence was not explicit or systematic. In particular, the systematic use of research-based evidence was not the norm. Therefore, the achievement of effective clinical practice through the implementation of guidelines, protocols and standards based on the best available evidence, was rather a hit-and-miss affair.

The clinical effectiveness initiative aims to change this such that when people are developing guidelines, protocols and standards they make more and better use of research-based evidence when it exists, combined appropriately with clinical expertise and patients' values and preferences, in an explicit and systematic process. Since clinical audit is one of the main vehicles for implementing guidelines, protocols or standards into everyday practice, if these are properly evidence-based and if clinical audit is successful in achieving changes in practice, then clinical audit has the potential to assist in the achievement of evidence-based practice.

A newly focused clinical audit cycle, referred to as the evidence-based clinical audit cycle, is illustrated in Figure 9.2. You will notice that the

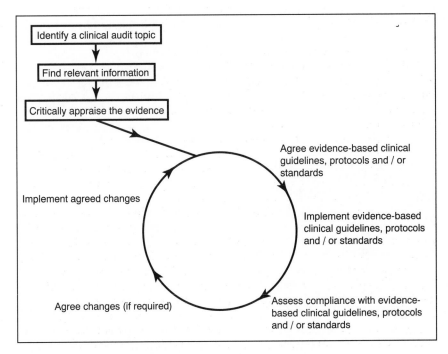

Figure 9.2 Evidence-based clinical audit cycle.

stages of the evidence-based clinical audit cycle are virtually identical to the clinical audit cycle that preceded it.

In practical terms, the main difference between the clinical audit cycles in Figures 9.1 and 9.2 is the emphasis on the evidence base in the latter. Skills already dealt with in this book, those of finding the evidence and critical appraisal, will be needed in order to take a systematic approach to identifying the evidence base.

The final point to make here is that while clinical audit is used to achieve evidence-based practice, with its focus on clinical interventions, it can only do this by also paying attention to the organizational environment within which clinical practice takes place. As already discussed in Chapters 2 and 8, changes to the organizational environment are often needed if individual practitioners are to be able to practise effectively according to the best available evidence. Therefore, many of the guidelines, protocols or standards that are agreed and implemented as part of the local clinical audit process include statements about the organizational environment. Clinical audit concerns itself with systems of care delivery as well as with clinical interventions.

Resources to support clinical audit

Since 1990, the Department of Health has invested about £50 million each year to support clinical audit (Buttery et al, 1994). This investment has led to the existence of a new cadre of staff with expertise in clinical audit: clinical audit staff. Many of these staff now also support activities relating to clinical effectiveness and evidence-based practice.

Clinical effectiveness and audit staff are employed in primary and acute care. Indeed, most trusts have a clinical effectiveness and/or clinical audit department. You are advised to find out what support is available locally. Clinical effectiveness and clinical audit staff may provide training in audit and may support any or all aspects of the clinical audit process. They might, for example, help you to:

- Identify topics for clinical audit
- Find relevant evidence
- Critically appraise evidence
- Facilitate the process of adapting national clinical guidelines
- Facilitate the development of local clinical guidelines, protocols or standards
- Design clinical audit projects
- Collect and analyse data
- Present clinical audit findings (written and verbal)
- Facilitate the development of action plans
- Follow up agreed changes.

Additionally, advice and support for clinical audit is available nationally from organizations such as professional bodies and the National Centre for Clinical Audit.

The importance of teams in effective clinical audit

Theoretically, it is possible for individual clinicians to undertake clinical audit alone. That is to say, it is possible for an individual to make explicit statements about expected practice performance, for example, by adopting the recommendations made in a national clinical guideline or by accepting a standard set by a professional organization. The individual would then measure his or her own compliance with those statements and then go on to change his or her behaviour to improve compliance if this proves necessary. However, clinical audit is a method that lends itself much more readily to groups of individuals wishing to generate changes in individuals' and collective practice.

A step-by-step approach to clinical audit

Identifying a topic

Before you can get on to the clinical audit cycle, a topic needs to be identified. Although obvious and, on the face of it, simple, in practice it is not always easy to identify important topics for clinical audit. Probably the commonest method used to identify potential topics is to brainstorm ideas, but this can sometimes result in the identification of only a few random potential topics for clinical audit. Perhaps more important than the number of potential topics identified is their importance in terms of potential for quality improvement.

It is common for topics to be identified which are *interesting* for one reason or another. It is unfortunately less usual for **common** areas of practice to be identified, where potential for improvement is greater due to the larger number of patients affected. Topics that relate to **unpopular** areas of practice are also often avoided, even though this may be due to unexplained variations in practice or uncertainties. There may be known problems in clinical or organizational systems, exploration of which through clinical audit will have a good chance of leading to improvements for patients and professionals. There are relatively limited resources available to support the clinical audit process, particularly professionals' time, so it is important that the choice of topic maximizes the impact of any clinical audit activity.

There are a number of tools available to assist you in identifying important topics. One method, **quality impact analysis**, is described below. In addition, patients and other service users are a good source of ideas for important and relevant topics for clinical audit. Their involvement in the clinical audit process is currently under-utilized (Kelson, 1995).

Quality impact analysis
Quality impact analysis (Healthcare Quality Quest, 1997) is a method of topic identification and prioritization. It offers a systematic way of

identifying possible topics for clinical audit which increases the number of topics suggested and identifies the degree of potential for quality improvement. It is best undertaken in groups since usually a number of heads are better than one for generating ideas! Quality impact analysis focuses on four categories of practice:

1. Areas where there has been some new research or development (including, for example, the appearance of a new national clinical guideline or standard).
2. Areas that are known to be problematic.
3. Areas that carry a high risk.
4. Areas that are high-volume (i.e. common activities).

The four categories are not mutually exclusive. Indeed, in quality impact analysis, it is common for one topic to fall into multiple categories. If this is the case, it is not especially important to which area the topic is assigned. The important thing is to consider a wide range of practice and service issues when trying to identify topics that may become the subject of clinical audit, and to select topics that have the greatest potential to benefit patients.

By identifying a list of potential topics in such a systematic way, the common situation of taking the first topic that comes to mind, as the topic for clinical audit, is avoided.

Once a number of potential topics have been identified, the next step is to prioritize them. Quality impact analysis is neither an exact nor a scientific process. However, it does provide one method for being explicit and systematic about the process of prioritization. You will see from Figure 9.3 that each potential topic is given a score on three dimensions: problems, risk and frequency. On each dimension, a score of 1 (low), 2 (medium) or 3 (high) is assigned. These scores are then added together to get a total score for each potential topic (maximum score 9). The total scores for each topic are then taken into account when selecting a topic for clinical audit. Usually, topics selected for clinical audit are those which have been assigned the highest scores.

In the example shown in Figure 9.3, a group of physiotherapists undertook a quality impact analysis to identify an important topic for clinical audit. The group identified one topic about which there is some new research or development: the management of acute low back pain (Royal College of General Practitioners, 1996). They assigned this topic a score of 3 for frequency, since acute low back pain forms a large part of their work, 3 for risk, since the risk associated with poor management is high, and a score of 3 for problems, since they know that variations in practice exist in this area. The total score assigned to the topic was 9 (the maximum possible).

Two topics were identified which they know to be associated with problems: patients failing to attend for planned appointments and long waiting lists. The total score assigned was 7 for both topics.

One topic was identified under the topic of high risk if incorrect: home visits. The total score assigned to the topic was 5.

Two topics were identified that relate to areas of practice which are

Think about your clinical practice and the services you provide. List up to three areas in each of the categories below and then score them (1 = low, 2 = medium, 3 = high) for problems, risk and frequency.

Area of work	freq	+ risk	+ probs	= Total
New research or developments:				
1. Management of acute low back pain	3	3	3	9
2.				
3.				
Known problems:				
1. Patients who do not attend	3	1	3	7
2. Waiting lists	3	1	3	7
3.				
High risk if incorrect:				
1. Home visits	1	3	1	5
2.				
3.				
Most frequent:				
1. Communication	3	2	3	8
2. Documentation	3	2	3	8
3.				

Figure 9.3 An example of a quality impact analysis.

high-volume: communication (total score assigned was 8) and documentation (total score assigned was also 8).

Patients' and users' views
As already stated, using patients' or users' views as a source of ideas for clinical audit topics is under-utilized (Kelson, 1995). However, patients' and users' views can be a particularly important source of topics. They are best placed to say what is important and relevant and, indeed, what is causing problems in the delivery of particular clinical services.

Chapter 5 describes in detail some of the formal approaches available to involve patients and users, including patient satisfaction surveys, meetings, stakeholder conferences, focus groups and citizens' juries. These are all approaches that can be used directly or indirectly in the context of clinical audit.

A further source of ideas for clinical audit, often overlooked, is patients' formal and informal complaints. While these undoubtedly form just the tip of the iceberg of failures in the healthcare system, every complaint can provide rich clues as to which areas of practice are most in need of some aspect of improvement. If trends in patients' complaints are apparent, then these areas also will be fruitful as topics for audit, in terms of offering potential for quality improvement.

Setting objectives for a clinical audit project

Once a topic has been identified, the next step is to set some objectives. At this stage they need only be broad, but it is critical that objectives appropriate to clinical audit are set. As you will see later, when you progress to the stage of agreeing explicit statements of best practice and developing criteria for assessing performance, the objectives will need to be refined.

When setting objectives for a clinical audit topic, it is useful to keep in mind a number of verbs which could be described as **audit verbs** (Williams, personal communication). Note that these verbs are all action verbs.

Audit verbs
- To improve
- To enhance
- To ensure
- To change.

Keeping these verbs in mind when setting objectives will help you to avoid falling into the trap of setting objectives which are not appropriate for clinical audit (a common problem). People often set objectives for clinical audit which are actually research objectives. This leads to a situation where a clinical audit project is neither a good clinical audit project nor a good research project. With this pitfall in mind, it is a good idea to be aware of some of the verbs that could be described as **research verbs** (Williams, personal communication):

Research verbs
- To identify
- To determine
- To discover.

In the example, shown in Figure 9.3, the topic selected was the management of acute low back pain. The audit process for this project is described throughout this section in the boxed text.

Agreeing guidelines, protocols or standards

As discussed earlier, guidelines, protocols and standards all provide explicit statements of best clinical practice or, in other words, provide explicit statements of expected practice performance. These are essential to the clinical audit process since, if there are no explicit statements

> The objective set by the group of physiotherapists was to improve the management of and documentation relating to patients with acute low back pain.

defining what is best practice, it becomes very difficult to measure if best practice is actually being achieved.

The idea that best clinical practice can be defined explicitly is not without its critics. They argue that every patient is an individual. The job of professionals, therefore, is to make clinical judgements about the interventions required for each individual to meet whatever goal has been set for or with them. There is therefore no place for explicit definitions of best clinical practice that relate to **groups** of patients.

In contrast, those who favour explicit definitions of best clinical practice accept that while of course individual patients will vary, there are many instances when it is entirely possible to anticipate the flow of events for a patient with a particular disease or condition. This process can be defined explicitly in the form of statements about what, and how, care is provided.

There is some strong empirical support for this view. Patients who present with very similar signs and symptoms can be treated in a variety of ways, depending on who they see and where they are seen (Gray et al, 1997). While some of this variation is to be expected, much of it appears to have no reasonable explanation and is unlikely to be rational, ethical or appropriate to the delivery of consistent, effective care.

The production of explicit definitions of best clinical practice, whatever form they take, represents an attempt to reduce these unjustified variations and, as such, should be welcomed. Furthermore, if these statements are based on the best available evidence, then achieving greater uniformity of practice will simultaneously ensure that practice will more consistently benefit patients.

If you accept the need for explicit definitions of best clinical practice then you can also accept that clinical audit enables the measurement of compliance with such definitions.

There are occasions when guidelines, protocols or standards are already available relating to a topic selected for clinical audit. If guidelines, protocols or standards already exist, it is important to assess them critically to check that they are up-to-date and to see if they are based on the best available evidence (see Chapters 7 and 8). When using guidelines, protocols or standards developed outside your local context, you will need to consider adapting them to ensure their local relevance (see Chapter 8).

It is common, however, to find that guidelines, protocols or standards do not exist. When faced with this situation, you and your colleagues will need to develop your own explicit statements of best clinical practice. This poses a dilemma, however, since only rarely will it be possible to go through the rigorous process described in the previous chapter. You will therefore have to take a pragmatic approach, since doing nothing is not an option if the topic is an important area of practice.

The first thing to do is to track down the most relevant research-based evidence (see Chapter 6) and some of the less robust evidence. This might include information about recognized good practice, through contact with your professional body or by accessing databases of practice and service developments. Librarians, clinical effectiveness and clinical audit staff will be able to help. The second thing to do will be to appraise the evidence you have collected (see Chapter 7). Once you have appraised the evidence and decided what is valid and relevant, you will need to combine this with evidence derived from your own clinical expertise and from patients.

A situation that you will often encounter is one where you find there is a virtual absence of good-quality research-based evidence. At least you can be assured that you will not fall into the trap of making explicit statements of best practice that do not accord with evidence from research! As a group, you will then need to draw confidently on the available clinical expertise to determine what is best practice, in the knowledge that this is the best available evidence. Expertise should, in these circumstances, be drawn from recognized centres of excellence as well as local expertise.

It is of course important to review all guidelines, protocols and standards regularly and, if new evidence relevant to the topic in question is produced, the guideline, protocol or standard must be amended to reflect this (NHSE, 1996b).

Implementing guidelines, protocols or standards

Achieving the successful implementation of guidelines, protocols or standards has proved problematic (Buttery et al, 1995). This is perhaps not surprising given that changes in behaviour are notoriously difficult to achieve (Rogers, 1983; Grol, 1992; Stocking, 1992; Wensing and Grol, 1994; Freemantle et al, 1995; Oxman et al, 1995).

A number of obstacles operating at the level of the individual and of the team can get in the way of successful implementation of guidelines, protocols and standards. Some of these are:

- An individual thinks he or she lacks the knowledge or ability to implement guidelines (Bandura, 1986, 1989)
- An individual thinks his or her performance is adequate (Prochaska and DiClemente, 1986)
- An individual denies any evidence demonstrating his or her poor performance (Parkes, 1978)
- An individual perceives the source of guidelines as not reputable (Hovland and Weiss, 1951; Turner, 1991)
- Team members individually assume that others will implement the change (Latane, 1981)
- A powerful subgroup within a team may resist change, making the less powerful majority feel obliged not to change either (Festinger, 1954)
- Good team spirit combined with a strong belief that care is excellent stifles disagreement with the prevailing view because of a desire to maintain the team spirit (Janis, 1982).

Taking into account the various obstacles that get in the way of implementing guidelines, protocols or standards and the lessons offered by a wide range of change theories, an appropriate strategy for implementing guidelines, protocols or standards will be a multifaceted one (Oxman et al, 1995). Such an implementation strategy might include:

- Mechanisms for involving a wide range of people in developing guidelines, protocols or standards (Robertson et al, 1996)
- The provision of training and positive feedback (Oxman et al, 1995)
- Feedback of poor performance (Robertson et al, 1996)
- Peer review (Grol, 1994; Robertson et al, 1996)
- The promotion of guidelines, protocols or standards by recognized opinion leaders (Hovland and Weiss, 1951; Turner, 1991)
- The allocation of responsibilities to specific team members (Latane, 1981)
- Ensuring that all subgroups in a team have equal influence (Festinger, 1954)
- Involving respected outsiders or managers (Janis, 1982).

Other chapters in this book provide more detailed discussion about what works in terms of change management (Chapter 3), getting research into practice (Chapter 4), and how to implement clinical guidelines (Chapter 8).

Assessing compliance with guidelines, protocols or standards

After implementing guidelines, protocols or standards, all of which comprise explicit statements of expected practice performance, the next step is to assess compliance with them. Such an assessment is necessary for two main reasons:

- In order that objective measurements can be made about the extent to which a guideline, protocol or standard has been successfully implemented into everyday clinical practice
- To identify reasons for non-compliance and, subsequently, to inform decisions about how to increase compliance.

There are a number of approaches to the assessment of compliance with a guideline, protocol or standard. **Criterion-based audit** is the most commonly used approach in the UK, although its origins are in the USA (Lembke, 1956, 1967). It can be used whether the explicit statements of best clinical practice take the form of a guideline, protocol or standard.

Criterion-based audit

Criterion-based audit is founded on the principle that it is possible to devise measurable criteria against which a valid, reliable and quantitative assessment of individuals' and groups' performance can be made in relation to a specific guideline, protocol or standard (Healthcare Quality Quest, 1997). The main characteristics of criterion-based audit are:

- A **compliance target** is set for each audit criterion, expressed as a percentage. These targets are sometimes referred to as standards, but

> **Example of criterion-based audit**
>
> Standard:
> Elderly people will be assessed for their risk of falling and provided with hip protectors as appropriate.
>
> Criterion 1:
> A risk assessment is carried out within 24 hours of admission to the elderly care ward.
>
> Compliance target:
> 90 per cent.
>
> Criterion 2:
> Patients at risk of falling will wear hip protectors.
>
> Complience target:
> 75 per cent.

should not be confused with the meaning of the word 'standards' used in this chapter as explicit statements of best practice

- Performance of **actual practice** is measured against each audit criterion, and calculated as a percentage (**compliance target**), making it possible to judge the extent to which an individual's or team's practice complies with the criterion
- Cases that do not comply with each audit criterion are subjected to further scrutiny to ascertain the reasons for non-compliance. From this, actions designed to improve compliance can be identified.

Indicator-based audit

Indicator-based audit is an extension of criterion-based audit (Jacobs and Dixon, 1975; Healthcare Quality Quest, 1997). The main differences are:

- Audit criteria are referred to as **aspects of care**, but will still be statements against which performance can be measured
- Compliance targets are referred to as **screening percentages**
- **Exceptions** to each aspect of care (audit criteria) are defined before any data are collected and excluded from the denominator when calculating percentage compliance with the relevant aspect of care (audit criteria)
- Screening percentages are therefore always set at 100 per cent or 0 per cent
- Since exceptions to each aspect of care (audit criteria) are excluded from the analysis, only cases not complying with a particular aspect of care (audit criteria) for reasons not defined before the data collection process, are subjected to further scrutiny. This usually takes the form of peer review to ascertain the reasons for non-compliance.

The following section will describe how to go about undertaking indicator-based audit rather than the more commonly used criterion-based audit. The former offers advantages, through setting screening percentages at 100 per cent or 0 per cent with specified exceptions, as opposed to setting less clearly defined and arbitrarily estimated compliance targets of, say, 90 per cent or 5 per cent.

Indicator-based audit provides a clearer platform from which to identify, and then deal with, problems resulting in a failure to meet the standard. You will see that this rules out the possibility of missing serious problems.

Developing audit indicators

Before an assessment can be made of compliance with guidelines, protocols or standards, the statements about what and how patient care should be provided, must first be converted into statements that specify how to **assess** what care is provided and how it is provided. This can be achieved through the development of audit indicators. An audit indicator has four parts (Healthcare Quality Quest, 1997):

1. The **aspect of care** being measured (the **audit criteria**). This states the evidence that would satisfy a professional that a particular dimension or feature of patient care or service is being provided.

Example of indicator-based audit

Standard:
  Elderly people will be assessed for their risk of falling and provided with hip protectors as appropriate.

Aspect of care 1:
  A risk assessment is carried out within 24 hours of admission to the elderly care ward.

Exceptions:
  None.

Screening per cent:
  100 per cent.

Aspect of care 2:
  Patients at risk of falling will wear hip protectors.

Exceptions:
  Patient refuses.

Screening percentage:
  100 per cent.

---

2. The **screening percentage** (sometimes referred to as a target or standard). This states the percentage of cases which are expected to conform to a particular aspect of care. When aspects of care (audit criteria) are events that are always expected, the screening percentage will normally be set at 100 per cent. In contrast, when an aspect of care is never expected, the screening percentage will normally be set at 0 per cent. While these screening percentages may appear challenging, they are very useful in so far as serious problems relating to individuals will not be missed.

By contrast, with criterion-based audit (see previous section), if a screening percentage is estimated at a level of, say, 95 per cent (allowing 5 per cent for justifiable exceptions), there is a danger that serious problems relating to individual cases might be hidden within this 5 per cent. It is not going to be clear what happened in the 5 per cent of cases of non-compliance. Were they instances that were unavoidable, for example because a patient chose not to comply, or was it due to a systems or practice performance failure? The problem is that it is all too easy to dismiss the failures as a proportion that you would expect not to comply. But a **single** system or practice performance failure is one too many, and one from which lessons need to be learned to avoid that particular failure in the future.

3. A preferable option, then, is to define known and acceptable **exceptions**. It is entirely appropriate to define exceptions to a particular aspect of care. By doing so, cases that fail to conform to an aspect of care for agreed, recognized and acceptable reasons, will not have an adverse effect on the overall assessment of compliance, since exceptions are removed from the denominator in these calculations. However, it is important to guard against including excuses for non-compliance as exceptions, since it is only by identifying problems that appropriate remedial action can be taken.

4. **Definitions and instructions** are needed to assist the data collection process. Sufficient detail is required so that the person(s) collecting the data know what they are looking for and where to find it. Indeed, the amount of detail included should enable someone different to collect the required data in future, when going around the cycle again.

Table 9.1 illustrates the process through an example of some standards relating to the management of acute low back pain and the audit indicators that were developed to enable compliance with these standards to be assessed.

Selecting an appropriate audit sample
There is no rule that states exactly how many cases is an appropriate number but, since the findings of audit are not generalizable to subjects outside the sample, large numbers are not normally needed. Indeed, if a large sample is being studied, you should question whether the purpose of the project is appropriate for clinical audit.

Usually, an appropriate sample size will be between 20 and 100 cases.

> The sample comprised the first three cases of acute low back pain discharged from a community trust during September 1996 for each physiotherapist (72 cases in total).

Table 9.1 Extracts of standards and audit indicators for a clinical audit project to improve the management of acute low back pain

Objective: to improve the management of patients with acute low back pain

Standard	Aspect of care (audit criteria)	Screening %	Exceptions	Definitions and instructions for data retrieval
1. A clinical diagnosis will be made at the end of the initial assessment	1(a) A clinical diagnosis will be recorded at the end of the assessment	100%	None	Physiotherapy notes
	1(b) The recorded clinical diagnosis will correspond with the department's diagnostic list	100%	None	Physiotherapy notes Diagnostic list
2. Measures of functional outcome will be used appropriately	2(a) A functional outcome measure will be recorded at the beginning of the intervention period	100%	None	Physiotherapy notes
	2(b) The same functional outcome measure will be used and recorded at the end of the intervention period	100%	None	Physiotherapy notes
3. Manipulation will be considered following assessment for patients with acute low back pain of less than six weeks duration[1]	3. Assessment includes suitability for manipulation	100%	3(a) Patients with osteoporosis 3(b) Presence of severe or progressive neurological deficit[2] 3(c) Patient declines manipulation	Physiotherapy notes
4. Rehabilitation will include appropriate information to facilitate self-management	4(a) A record is made of advice given on exercises to promote self-management	100%	None	Physiotherapy notes
	4(b) A record is made of information leaflet(s) on self-management given to patients	100%	None	Physiotherapy notes

[1] There is strong evidence that manipulation is effective within the first six weeks of onset of acute or recurrent low back pain (*Clinical Guidelines for the Management of Acute Low Back Pain*, Royal College of General Practitioners, 1996)

[2] There is evidence to suggest that manipulation is contraindicated in view of the risk of neurological complications (*Clinical Guidelines for the Management of Acute Low Back Pain*, Royal College of General Practitioners, 1996)

The important points to remember are:

- The audit sample should include subjects who have something in common that relates directly to the aspects of care being assessed
- Consideration should be given to whether any cases ought to be specifically excluded, e.g. the very old, the very young, and so on
- Data must be retrievable for all cases identified for inclusion in the sample
- Consideration should be given to the time period of the data collection phase of the audit cycle to take account of, for example, seasonal variations
- The number of cases included in the sample should be large enough for you to feel confident that the observed level of compliance and any associated problems provide a reasonable reflection of reality.

In situations where there are only small total numbers of cases, for example, because the condition or practice is rare, it is possible to include the entire population in the study. This removes any of the problems of selecting an appropriate sample size.

Other methodological issues

- **Statistical analysis versus professional judgement in determining whether performance is acceptable**. By using absolute screening percentages (i.e. 100 per cent or 0 per cent) in combination with defined exceptions (as opposed to stating compliance targets that are not absolute), the estimation of statistically significant deviations away from expected levels of compliance is not particularly important. If expected compliance is absolute, then **any** deviation may be significant. Whether or not an observed variation away from the expected absolute screening percentage is significant is a matter for discussion and judgement. The professionals themselves must decide how clinically significant a particular level of compliance or deviation is.
- **Detecting changes in performance over time**. While it is possible to calculate sample sizes that will ensure that an audit sample is of sufficient size to detect a robust and a clinically significant change over time in levels of compliance with a guideline, protocol or standard (Altman, 1991), this will usually require relatively large samples. However, an alternative approach to detecting changes in compliance levels is to observe trends in compliance with a particular guideline, protocol or standard over time (Barton and Thompson, 1993). This will require you to make a number of revolutions of the audit cycle. This is desirable for a number of reasons, discussed later, and need not be onerous if the sample size is small.
- **Attributing change to the clinical audit process: a warning**. It is especially important to remember that even if an audit sample is large enough to demonstrate a statistically significant improvement in compliance with a guideline, protocol or standard over time, this improvement cannot be attributed definitively to the audit process. Attribution of change to the clinical audit process (or to anything else)

> - All subjects in the sample had acute low back pain in common. It would not have been appropriate, for example, to include patients with cervical pain
> - All cases were eligible for inclusion in the sample since the standards were considered to be applicable to all patients with acute low back pain
> - Data were retrieved for all 72 subjects who comprised the sample
> - The time period that yielded the sample for the audit was considered not atypical of any other time period that could have been selected
> - The number of cases included in the sample was considered large enough to reasonably reflect reality.

is possible only by conducting some form of controlled study. In the context of clinical audit, it is improvement itself that is most important, not precisely what caused the improvement (although it would be very nice to know!). Determining what **actions** are required to generate **improvements** in compliance is, however, critical.

Collecting data

What to collect and where to find it. Exactly which data is required will depend on the audit indicators. The definitions and instructions component of the audit indicator will tell the person(s) collecting the data what the data required looks like and where to find it.

When the data required is collected routinely, either in patient records or in some other source, data collection may be **retrospective** (collected some time after the information was routinely recorded) or **concurrent** (collected at the same time as the information is being routinely recorded).

When the data required is not collected routinely, it will be necessary to agree a system whereby professionals record additional information for the duration of the data collection phase of the clinical audit cycle. This approach to data collection is referred to as **prospective** since special arrangements have to be made for additional information to be recorded.

Whichever data is collected, it is important that it is anonymous, as discussed shortly, with issues of confidentiality. This will require a master index to be kept, indicating which case is which, but the individual audit records should not contain information that allows individual patients to be identified. Rather, each case should be given a number which allows you to identify which case it is by referring to your master index. Once the audit project is completed, the master index and the audit records should be shredded.

> The data was collected retrospectively from patients' notes, using a checklist.

Who collects the data? This will depend on the local context and on available resources. It may be possible for a member of the clinical audit staff, if available, to collect the data for you. While this will save time, it will not help to achieve a sense of ownership among the professionals involved. To increase ownership, or to share the workload in the absence of clinical audit staff, it might be possible to divide the total number of cases that comprise the audit sample between a number of individual practitioners.

When data collection is prospective, the load can be shared even further, so that each individual practitioner collects data for his or her own cases, using a specially developed checklist.

> One physiotherapist collected the data for all seventy-two subjects that comprised the sample.

Before undertaking the data collection and analysis for any project, it is of the utmost importance to undertake a pilot study, of just five or so cases, to check that:

- The data can be found where you anticipated it would be
- You have not missed out anything important
- The person collecting the data understands your definitions and instructions.

Time invested at this stage is always well worth it and will save tears later!

Analysing clinical audit data

If samples are very small and few data items are collected, it is feasible to analyse the data using only a pen and paper, and perhaps a calculator to calculate percentage conformance with each aspect of care. Usually, though, you will need access to a computer which is loaded with some sort of database or spreadsheet package. Once the data is entered, very simple manipulations will calculate percentage conformance with each aspect of care. For the reasons outlined earlier, more advanced statistical techniques are rarely required.

> A software package called Statistical Package for the Social Sciences (SPSS) was used for data analysis. This was undertaken by clinical audit staff.

Feedback of audit findings

It is useful to distinguish between audit findings and audit results. Audit **findings** refer to levels of compliance with guidelines, protocols and standards, as measured through audit indicators. Other observations made during the data collection process which might inform discussions about the problems associated with lack of compliance and their possible solutions, might also constitute audit findings. In contrast, audit **results** refer to **changes, improvements, impacts and benefits**, occurring as a result of the clinical audit process. Understanding the distinction between these two terms is important. Keeping in mind the description of audit results helps to maintain the momentum of clinical audit projects after data has been analysed and fed back.

At this stage, it is worth reiterating that the intention of the feedback process is to identify where improvements are required and what actions might lead to those improvements. It should not be a punitive exercise. It is therefore wise to agree the reporting mechanisms and format of the feedback before any data collection or analysis takes place. By doing this, everyone will be clear from the outset whether findings will be presented at the level of the whole organization, team or individual practitioner.

Feedback of audit findings is best undertaken in both verbal and written forms. Normally, a meeting involving all relevant stakeholders should be organized, at which audit findings (in the format already agreed) can be fed back and discussed. Before this meeting, an initial report should be drafted, which will be finalized after the findings have been fed back and discussed. The following could be used as a template for an audit report:

- Background to the clinical audit project/project rationale
- Project aims and objectives
- Guidelines, protocols or standards
- Audit indicators (includes aspects of care/audit criteria)
- Methodology
- Audit findings
- Details about how the audit findings have been fed back (for completion after feedback and discussion)

Compliance with each aspect of care (see Table 9.1) was presented at the overall level, the level of teams and the level of the individual physiotherapist, maintaining confidentiality of individuals' performance.

A draft report was produced by a member of clinical audit staff in close liaison with the audit project lead. The draft report was then distributed to all physiotherapists ahead of a preplanned audit meeting.

The audit findings were presented by the audit project lead and a member of the clinical audit staff at the preplanned audit meeting, attended by the therapy services manager and all physiotherapists. The audit meeting also provided an opportunity for reinforcing the importance of the standards already agreed.

After the meeting, the audit report was updated to include details of the action plan agreed, plans for re-audit and the changes, benefits and impacts generated by the audit thus far.

- Action plan (for completion after feedback and discussion)
- Changes, benefits or impacts generated by the audit activity (to be completed after discussion of audit findings and to be updated as progress is made with the action plan)
- Plans for re-audit (to be completed after discussion of the audit findings).

When feeding back audit findings, it is important to use a variety of methods of presentation to account for the fact that people respond differently to different methods. For example, some people feel most comfortable with words, while others respond better to tabular presentations and still others prefer graphical presentations.

Additionally, it is important to present audit findings at a variety of levels of aggregation: overall compliance; compliance at the level of, for example, locality or team (possibly made anonymous so that the performance of a particular locality or team is only known to its members); and the level of the individual, which must be made anonymous so that only the individual practitioner can recognize his or her own performance in relation to others. If only overall levels of compliance are presented, it is easy for individual practitioners or groups of practitioners to assume that any non-compliance is the fault of other individuals or groups.

Confidentiality

The results of clinical audit, that is, the changes, improvements, impacts and benefits generated, should be made widely available to practitioners, managers and the public. However, clinical audit findings (i.e. levels of compliance with guidelines, protocols or standards), will usually remain confidential at the level of individual patient and practitioner. This is important since, while clinical audit may uncover performance that falls short of that expected, open discussion and resolution of problems is gained through uninhibited participation in clinical audit (British Medical Association Clinical Audit Committee, 1996; Womack et al, 1997).

Individual trusts may have confidentiality policies relating to clinical audit, and advice should be sought from your clinical effectiveness and audit department and/or your professional organization before embarking on clinical audit.

Agreeing changes (if required)

If careful consideration has been given to the selection of a topic for clinical audit, it is very likely that changes will be required. This is so for two main reasons.

1. In order to maximize the impact of clinical audit, areas of practice that are known to already accord with best practice will have been avoided. While it may be tempting to select areas such as these, one should question the motivation for selecting areas not needing

improvement when there are many other areas of practice where improvements are needed.

2. If new or modified evidence-based guidelines, protocols or standards have been developed or adapted as part of the clinical audit process, which differ from current practice, it is unlikely that, in the short term, compliance will be complete since, as discussed earlier, achieving changes in behaviour is complex and very difficult to achieve. The expectation will normally be that some changes will be required before compliance with guidelines, protocols or standards is achieved completely.

A very common pitfall in the clinical audit process is to stop after the measurement of compliance with a guideline, protocol or standard. However, great efforts should be made to ensure that the clinical audit process does not falter at this stage. If it does, not only will the activity to that point constitute a waste of resources, but the process will fail to ensure that guidelines, protocols or standards are implemented into everyday practice. An opportunity will then have been lost to achieve evidence-based and more effective practice.

Agreeing required changes demands a substantial amount of discussion. This discussion should be informed by any observations of problems noted during data collection and should also be informed by the peer-review process conducted around cases not conforming to various aspects of care.

While the use of aspects of care (audit criteria) can take some of the subjectivity out of this process, it nevertheless requires judgements to be made about:

- Which aspects of performance need to be improved
- What actions are needed to generate improvements in performance.

It is important that all disciplines required to take action are involved in these discussions. If this does not happen, it is very unlikely that members of the disciplines required to take action, but who have not been party to the discussions or agreements, will pay attention to requests for their cooperation. Clearly, this will result in failure to achieve agreed actions and, subsequently, failure to achieve improvements in performance.

Once agreement has been reached about what changes are required, an action plan must be produced assigning responsibility to specific individuals, together with expected time scales.

> During the audit meeting, at which the audit findings were fed back and discussed, it was agreed that improvements were required and that re-audit would take place in 12 months' time. Each of the three team leaders was allocated responsibility to hold further discussions with his or her staff about how to achieve improvements with a view to demonstrating these in the next audit cycle.

Implementing agreed changes

The successful implementation of agreed actions requires that professionals change their behaviour. Given that the obstacles to successful implementation of agreed changes are likely to be similar to those which get in the way of implementing guidelines, protocols and standards, it seems logical that the multifaceted strategy suggested earlier in this chapter for implementing guidelines, protocols or standards will, to a large extent, be equally applicable in the context of implementing agreed changes. Strategies for change management are also described in Chapters 3, 4 and 8.

Going around the cycle again

Given the importance of each stage of the clinical audit cycle in contributing to the achievement of change, it might be surprising that clinical audit projects relatively infrequently make more than one revolution of the cycle (Buttery et al., 1995). If clinical audit is to be effective, more revolutions must become the norm. So, take note and make sure that clinical audit is truly a cyclical process leading to continuous improvements in quality.

This said, however, it is clear that going around the cycle with an ever-increasing number of topics will rapidly exhaust any resources available for audit! As with most other aspects of clinical audit, a pragmatic approach is needed to ensure that any programme of clinical audit is balanced in terms of undertaking new audit projects and undertaking a second or subsequent cycle.

One approach to this is to be selective about what and when to re-audit. Limiting re-audit to areas where there is poor compliance with particular aspects of care will reduce the size of the undertaking. When to undertake re-audit will depend on the circumstances of each clinical audit project. While it is, of course, necessary to wait until agreed actions have been implemented in accordance with the action plan, it is a good idea to repeat the data collection process as soon as possible. This will check that actions have indeed been taken and that these actions have had the desired effect in terms of increasing compliance with guidelines, protocols or standards. At the very least, it is necessary to repeat the assessment of compliance with a guideline, protocol or standard once, unless compliance was perfect or near perfect, in order to get some indication about whether compliance improves.

Summary

Clinical audit provides an apparently ideal mechanism for getting evidence into practice, thereby contributing to the enhancement of clinical practice and service delivery. If it is to be successful, however, it must generate changes in the clinical behaviour of professionals.

Achieving such change is known to be difficult, but by paying attention to **all** aspects of the clinical audit cycle and not focusing exclusively on the data collection and analysis phase of the cycle, assessing compliance with guidelines, protocols or standards, will help to ensure that clinical audit is successful in achieving change.

The whole clinical audit cycle, as described in this chapter, provides immense opportunity for putting into practice the many mechanisms which together can achieve change:

- Every stage of the clinical audit cycle provides opportunities for involving a wide range of people
- All stages of the clinical audit cycle allow for the delivery of training and positive feedback, sometimes formal and sometimes informal. In particular, this is possible when feeding back audit findings to those whose practice is the subject of the clinical audit process
- The feedback of audit findings stage of the clinical audit cycle provides an ideal opportunity to feedback information on poor performance, anonymously except to the individual(s) involved
- The stage of feedback of audit findings offers a clear opportunity for peer review of cases of non-compliance
- The stage of the clinical audit cycle when changes are agreed provides a perfect opportunity to assign responsibilities to specific team members
- By paying careful attention to the membership of the audit project team, it is possible to ensure that all subgroups are on an equal footing with one another
- It is possible to involve clinical audit staff or other outsiders to act as facilitators at any stage of the clinical audit cycle when discussions take place and/or agreements need to be reached.

Acknowledgments

Nancy Dixon, Nicola Johnson and Sarah McGeorge are thanked for their advice on this chapter.

Further reading

Crombie, I. K. (1993). *Audit Handbook: Improving Health Care Through Clinical Audit.* Wiley.

Dixon, N. (1996). *Good Practice in Clinical Audit. A Summary of Selected Literature to Support Criteria for Clinical Audit.* National Centre for Clinical Audit.

Grol, R. and Lawrence, M. (1995). *Quality Improvement by Peer Review.* Oxford University Press.

Healthcare Quality Quest (1997). *Getting Audit Right to Benefit Patients.* Healthcare Quality Quest.

Irvine, D. and Irvine, S. (1997). *Making Sense of Audit.* Radcliffe.

Kogan, M., Redfern, S., Kober, A., et al. (1995). *Making Use of Clinical Audit: A Guide to Practice in the Health Professions.* Open University Press.

Malby, R. (1995). *Clinical Audit for Nurses and Therapists.* Scutari.

National Health Service Management Executive (1994). *Getting Ahead with Clinical Audit: A Facilitator's Guide.* National Health Service Training Directorate.

References

Altman, D. (1991). *Practical Statistics for Medical Research*. Chapman & Hall.

Bandura, A. (1986). *Social Foundations of Thought and Action*. Sage.

Bandura, A. (1989). Perceived self-efficacy in the exercise of personal agency. *Psychologist*, **2**, 411–24.

Barton, A. and Thompson, R. G. (1993). Is audit bad research? *Audit Trends*, **1**(2), 41–53.

British Medical Association Clinical Audit Committee (1996). *Ethical Issues in Audit*. British Medical Association.

Buck, N., Devlin, H. B. and Lunn, J. N. (1987). *The Report of a Confidential Enquiry into Perioperative Deaths*. Nuffield Provincial Hospitals Trust and King's Fund.

Buttery, Y., Walshe, K., Coles. J. and Bennett J. (1994). *Evaluating Medical Audit: The Development of Audit*. CASPE Research.

Buttery, Y., Walshe, K., Rumsey, M., et al., (1995). *Evaluating Audit in England: a Review of Twenty Nine Programmes*. CASPE Research.

Chartered Society of Physiotherapy (1993). *Standards of Physiotherapy Practice*. Chartered Society of Physiotherapy.

College of Occupational Therapists (1990). *Guidelines for Documentation*. College of Occupational Therapists.

Department of Health (1989). *Working for Patients: Working Paper 6*. HMSO.

Department of Health (1991a). *Report on Confidential Enquiries into Maternal Deaths in the UK, 1985–87*. Department of Health.

Department of Health (1991b). PL/CNO (91/3). *Audit for the Nursing and Therapy Professions in HCHS: Allocation of Funds 1991/92*. Department of Health.

Festinger, L. (1954). A theory of social comparison processes. *Human Relations*, **7**, 117–40.

Fowkes, G. F. (1982). Medical audit cycle: a review of methods and research in clinical practice. *Med Educ*, **16**, 228–38.

Freemantle, N., Grilli, R., Grimshaw, J., et al. (1995). Implementing findings of medical research: the Cochrane Collaboration on Effective Professional Practice. *Qual Health Care*, **4**, 45–7.

Gray, J. A. M., Haynes, R. B., Sackett, D. L., et al. (1997). Transferring evidence from research into practice: 3. Developing evidence-based clinical policy. *Evidence Based Medicine*, **2**(2), 36–8.

Grol, R. (1992). Implementing guidelines in general practice care. *Qual Health Care*, **1**, 184–91.

Grol, R. (1994). Quality improvement by peer review in primary care: a practical guide. *Qual Health Care*, **3**, 147–52.

Healthcare Quality Quest (1997). *Getting Audit Right to Benefit Patients*. Healthcare Quality Quest.

Hovland, C. and Wess, W. (1951). The influence of source credibility on communication effectiveness. *Public Opin Q*, **15**, 635–50.

Jacobs, C. M. and Dixon, N. (1975). *Performance Evaluation Procedure for Auditing and Improving Patient Care. (PEP) Primer*. Joint Commission on Accreditation of Hospitals.

Janis, I. L. (1982). *Group Think: Psychological Studies of Policy Decisions and Fiascos*. Houghton Mifflin.

Kelson, M. (1995). *Consumer Involvement Initiatives in Clinical Audit and Outcomes: A Review of Developments and Issues in the Identification of Good Practice*. College of Health.

Latane, B. (1981). The psychology of social impact. *Am Psychol*, **36**, 343–56.

Lembke, P. A. (1956). Medical auditing by scientific methods. Illustrated by major female pelvic surgery. *JAMA*, **162**(7), 646–55.

Lembke, P. A. (1967). Evolution of medical audit. *JAMA*, **199**(8), 111–18.

NHS Executive (1996a). *Clinical Audit in the NHS. Using Clinical Audit in the NHS: A Position Statement*. Department of Health.

NHS Executive. (1996b). *Clinical Guidelines: Using Clinical Guidelines to Improve Patient Care Within the NHS*. Department of Health.

NHS Executive (1996c). *Promoting Clinical Effectiveness: A Framework for Action In and Through the NHS*. Department of Health.

NHS Management Executive (1994). EL(94)20. *Clinical Audit: 1994/95 and Beyond*. Department of Health.

Oxman, A., Thomson, M. A., Davis, D. A. and Haynes, R. B. (1995). No magic bullets: a systematic review of 102 trials of interventions to improve professional practice. *Can Med Assoc J*, **153**(10), 1423–31.

Parkes, C. M. (1978). *Bereavement: Studies of Grief in Adult Life*. Penguin.

Prochaska, J. O., and DiClemente, C. C. (1986). Towards a comprehensive model of change. In *Treating Addictive Behaviour: Processes of Change* (W. R. Miller and N. Heather, eds) pp. 33–62, Plenum Press.

Robertson, N., Baker, R. and Hearnshaw, H. (1996). Changing the clinical behaviour of doctors: a psychological framework. *Qual Health Care*, **5**, 51–4.

Rogers, E. (1983). *Diffusion of Innovations*. Free Press.

Royal College of General Practitioners (1996). *Clinical Guidelines for the Management of Acute Low Back Pain*. Royal College of General Practitioners.

Royal College of Nursing (1980). *Standards in Nursing*. Royal College of Nursing.

Royal College of Nursing (1981). *Towards Standards*. Royal College of Nursing.

Royal College of Physicians (1990). *Medical Audit: A First Report – What, Why and How?* Royal College of Physicians.

Royal College of Speech and Language Therapists (1996). *Communicating Quality*. Royal College of Speech and Language Therapists.

Royal College of Surgeons (1990). *Guidelines for Clinical Audit in Surgical Practice*. Royal College of Surgeons.

Stocking, B. (1992). Promoting change in clinical care. *Qual Health Care*, **1**, 56–60.

Turner, J. C. (1991). *Social Influence*. Open University Press.

Walshe, K. and Coles J. (1993). *Evaluating Audit: Developing a Framework*. CASPE Research.

Wensing, M. and Grol, R. (1994). Single and combined strategies for implementing changes in primary care: a literature review. *Int J Qual Health Care*, **6**, 115–32.

Womack, C., Roger, S., Lavin, M. (1997). Disclosure of clinical audit records in law: risks and possible defences. *BMJ*, **315**, 1369–70.

The Way Forwards

The previous chapters have provided you with a logical overview of evidence-based healthcare, the necessary skills and their application to achieve this. Key themes are apparent and these are brought together in this section to assist you in developing local action plans, making evidence-based healthcare happen.

Principles to guide you in achieving this are presented, recognizing that healthcare is changing constantly and policy initiatives continue to be developed. This creates a fluid environment in which to strive for improvements in healthcare. There is not one single way of doing this, but guiding principles allow for flexibility and adaptation depending on each situation.

Looking to the future, there is every indication that the emphasis on evidence-based healthcare and clinical effectiveness will continue to grow. What this means in terms of healthcare delivery is not clear cut, but it is important to act now with an eye to the future.

10
Making evidence-based healthcare happen

Judy Mead and Tracy Bury

Introduction

This final chapter provides you with an opportunity to recap on some of the key themes that have recurred throughout this book. It will consider how you can apply these in order to achieve evidence-based healthcare in your own setting, whether this is:

- With individual patients
- Managing and delivering therapy services
- Influencing those who commission or purchase therapy services.

Key questions are posed for therapists wanting to make evidence-based healthcare a reality in their individual practice or service. Healthcare continues to change and a look to the future tries to determine how evidence-based healthcare will develop in the context of health services in the UK. Will it survive or is it a fad? If it survives, will it be because of or in spite of politicians, health professionals and patients? Both challenges and opportunities for therapists will be highlighted.

Key themes

The preceding chapters have been arranged to help you take a logical, step-by-step approach to evidence-based healthcare. The introductory chapters set the scene and clarified terminology. The next section illustrated the importance of effective change management, including the influence that service users can have in facilitating change. Subsequent chapters discussed specific skills that are required to achieve evidence-based healthcare, and described ways in which evidence can be incorporated into practice, through clinical guidelines and clinical audit, to achieve quality improvement.

The key themes described in this chapter are those which are fundamental to the achievement of evidence-based healthcare, much of which has been the subject of emphasis in the preceding chapters. They are:

- Facilitating change
- Involving consumers
- Collaboration
- Information
- Continuing professional development
- Achieving quality improvement.

Facilitating change

There is not a chapter in this book that does not explicitly refer to, or imply the need for, change in order to successfully implement evidence-based healthcare. This can take many forms, for example:

- Changing your own clinical practice in the light of establishing the best available evidence
- Facilitating organizational change in a service-wide initiative
- Changing personal behaviour, for example, communicating more effectively with patients by involving them to a greater extent in decision-making about their care
- Developing new personal skills that will facilitate change, such as critical appraisal or leadership.

Evidence-based healthcare is an approach to quality improvement for which, by its very nature, change is fundamental. Nothing remains static. Knowledge changes all the time. Practitioners change through their own personal and professional development. They find themselves working with different groups of colleagues from their own and other backgrounds, and need to adapt accordingly. Each patient is an individual, with different values and experiences, even if the disease process is more predictable. Professionals therefore need to adapt to each patient's unique needs. Change is ever-present in clinical settings.

Managing, or being involved in, organizational change, is at least as challenging as individuals dealing with change. Organizational change requires planning, the involvement of all interested parties, a common understanding of the objectives, organizational commitment and sensitivity to the needs of others. Chapter 3 highlights the importance of individuals reflecting during a change process, in order to see and understand other perspectives as well as their own.

The rewards of successful change, in bringing about a greater degree of evidence-based healthcare, will be seen in improvements in both benefit (health gain) and quality of experience for patients and a greater confidence and satisfaction on the part of practitioners and purchasers, in achieving the best deal for patients.

Facilitating change: What can you do?

If you are involved in facilitating a change process:

- Is there a shared vision of where you want to get to (clear, agreed overall objectives)?
- Have all the key players (stakeholders) been involved at an early stage?
- Have you taken time to understand the individual needs of each of the stakeholders?
- Is there a shared understanding of the issues and a shared acceptance of the need for change?
- Are there clear step-by-step objectives/goals for change?
- Has there been adequate planning, and resources made available, e.g. time, support?
- Is there is genuine commitment to change, and the impact of change, from the organization?
- Have you provided yourself with opportunities to learn from the experience of others?
- Have you allowed all those involved in change time for reflection and consolidation?
- Do you have the necessary personal attributes to facilitate change?
- Have you considered using any of the tools and techniques described in Chapter 3?
- Have you considered the approaches to getting research into practice described in Chapter 4, for which there is some evidence of effectiveness?
- The use of clinical guidelines and clinical audit are likely to require personal and/or organizational change if they are to achieve quality improvement. Have you considered strategies for change management as part of these activities?

Involving consumers

The importance of involving consumers is highlighted in almost every chapter. The culture of patients as partners alongside professionals will not have been universally familiar. Where it is, there are challenges as well as rewards in applying the principles comprehensively. Where the culture is less embedded, personal change management strategies may be needed in order to achieve an approach based on sharing information and facilitating decision-making by patients. Empowering patients as partners in their care, and working together to achieve gains that will make real differences that matter to patients, will be a rewarding experience.

Consumers' perspectives in interpreting evidence of effectiveness and applying it to their lives will be very different from the perspectives of professionals (Chapter 5). The importance of involving consumers in developing relevant evidence-based patient information, developing clinical guidelines or identifying important topics for clinical audit programmes, is clear. For example, in developing clinical guidelines, the evidence may suggest a technique that is effective, but patient representatives may highlight this as being unacceptable, for example to a group of patients from a particular cultural background. In these circumstances, the guideline should highlight alternative models of care, which describe the benefits and risks of the options, to assist patients and health professionals in making decisions.

What can you do?

Chapter 5 includes useful **practice points**, which you are invited to revisit and apply. Meanwhile, consider the following:

- Have you asked colleagues to give you feedback on how you communicate with patients?
- Do you encourage patients to make decisions, or do you make them for patients? Do you give patients a choice?
- How much information do you write down for patients? Do you check to see how well patients remember and understand what you have told them?
- How familiar are you with local sources of health information?
- If your department produces patient information, is it based on up-to-date and reliable evidence? Did you involve patients in writing it? Does it answer questions that patients want answered?
- Do you welcome comments from patients about their treatment, or the information you provide?
- Have you ever invited patients to a departmental meeting?
- Do you belong to local patient groups?
- Have you asked patients how they judge the success of an episode of treatment?

Collaboration

Evidence-based healthcare has been described, particularly in the first two chapters of this book, as being a complex process requiring collaboration between practitioners, service users, managers, purchasers of healthcare and the general public. There is an interdependency between the needs of the population and the needs of individuals, in order to achieve the greatest benefit for finite resources, which can be informed by all relevant groups.

More specifically, evidence-based practice needs to be delivered by teams with common, patient-centred goals, within effective systems of care, where there are no tribal barriers, and where all parties contribute constructively to making the systems work better for patients. The effectiveness of one member of a multiprofessional team working in an evidence-based way will be influenced by the approach of other members of the team. It needs to be a collective effort to maximize patient benefit.

Having a common understanding of the language that has evolved alongside evidence-based healthcare and clinical effectiveness can considerably enhance the relationship between all concerned. Questions from those commissioning healthcare about the evidence of interventions/services should not be seen by providers as a threat, but as an opportunity to influence service provision to maximize efficiency and health gain.

Dealing with uncertainty due to large gaps in the research evidence reflects the reality of healthcare, but should not stifle a move to more evidence-based decision-making. However, these gaps need to be addressed. Everyone has a responsibility to influence the research agenda and commissioning process, in order to ensure accountability for money invested in research that fulfils service needs. Active collaboration between practitioners, managers and researchers is important in then taking forwards the required research.

Collaboration: What can you do?

- In making decisions with your patient(s) about their care, who else do you need to involve?
- Would there be advantages in having an interprofessional clinical audit programme?
- If you are developing local, evidence-based statements of best practice or implementing a national clinical guideline, who else do you need to involve?
- How can you help purchasers become more aware of the best available evidence for your services?
- How can you find out how to communicate most effectively with commissioners and purchasers? Who do you need to work with? What language and approach will they recognize and be able to respond to?
- How well do you know people you can influence, but also who can help? Is there an R&D coordinator in your trust? Do you know and use your local clinical audit/clinical effectiveness teams? Do you have a communication route to your local education consortium? Do you know who your regional director of R&D is? More importantly, do all these people know you?

Information

Evidence-based healthcare requires information. In the first place, information has to be about the evidence itself. It will need to be:

- Systematically gathered to ensure that important sources of information are not missed

- Critically appraised to ensure that the information applied in evidence-based healthcare is reliable and valid
- Inclusive of information derived from patients about their experience of care, their symptoms, their values and their individual needs.

Such information can be used to inform decisions about healthcare with individual patients, or it may form the evidence base for the development of nationally relevant clinical guidelines or locally derived, explicit statements of best practice.

Chapter 6 takes a step-by-step approach to finding the evidence. Fundamental is the need to identify a clear question by identifying the patient or population group, the intervention, the outcome and any alternative choices of intervention. Once a comprehensive literature search has been carried out, Chapter 7 provides detailed guidance on the critical appraisal of research papers you may have found. You will be able to determine whether or not you can trust what you read. If you can satisfy yourself that the research is reliable, you can then decide whether it is applicable to **your question**, whether it be about individual patients or services.

Information, in the form of clinical information, is also necessary in order to determine whether or not the evidence you are using in practice is benefiting patients. This might be by gathering clinical data that measures whether or not you are actually doing what your explicit statements of best practice (see Chapter 9) say you should be doing. For example, the *Clinical Practice Guideline on Splinting Adults with Neurological Dysfunction* (Association of Chartered Physiotherapists Interested in Neurology, 1998) states "The alignment of the limb within the splint should facilitate the functional re-education of the limb following the removal of the splint". Does this happen? How can such information be collected?

Such forms of measurement are about the process of care. Benefits to patients and resultant health gain can also be measured by the use of appropriate, validated outcome measures. These might be physical measures, such as strength, or measures assessed by patients themselves, for example about well-being, which can be used at the beginning and end of an episode of care to determine the degree of improvement in a reliable way. This book has not attempted to deal with the use of outcome measures. This is not because they are considered unimportant. Outcome measures form an important component for the assessment of the benefits resulting from evidence-based healthcare. However, there is a limited number of validated outcome measures relevant to therapists and a full discussion of the use of outcome measures would require a further book! Equally, some would argue that if processes are based on strong evidence of effectiveness, a beneficial outcome can be assumed and outcome measures are unnecessary. For therapists, such strong evidence is unlikely to be available, and more work on the development of outcome measures is needed. Patient assessed outcome measures are likely to be of particular value.

Information: What can you do?

- How familiar is your local health service librarian with your services?
- Does your library have the most relevant databases for you, your staff and services?
- Do you use the more specialist library sources housed with your professional body?
- Do you have at least one computer where you work which is easily accessible, with the Internet, databases and relevant mailbase/ discussion groups?
- If you are a manager, have you considered how staff working in isolated settings such as health centres and GP practices can access information?
- Have you tried journal clubs (see Chapter 7) or an in-service session to critically appraise literature relevant to a current clinical situation?
- Do you have a programme to collect data to evaluate elements of your service against agreed, explicit statements of best practice?
- Have you or your manager talked to your local education consortium or research and development directorate to press for funding to access better information?

Continuing professional development

Continuing professional development (CPD), or lifelong learning, is a necessary component for the successful application of every element of evidence-based healthcare described in this book. Change implies learning, simply by moving from one state to another, as described in Chapter 3. In addition, strategies for the introduction of change include the need for reflection and skill development. The development of skills and attributes to facilitate partnerships with patients and promote evidence-based patient choice (Chapter 5) may require personal as well as professional development. The development or enhancement of skills such as literature searching (Chapter 6), critical appraisal (Chapter 7), using clinical guidelines (Chapter 8) and the implementation of evidence through clinical audit (Chapter 9) will all be strengthened by being applied within a supportive, learning environment. Skills can then be developed and tried out, feedback on personal performance can be given constructively and openly, and time can be made available for reflecting on practice.

The challenge of CPD activity, however, must be the ability to demonstrate consequential benefit to patients, whether through their enhanced experience of care or in terms of health gain. The use of various educational approaches was discussed in Chapter 4, showing variable results. It is disappointing that few studies have focused on improvements in patient outcomes as opposed to practitioner behaviour. This was further supported in a study by Powell (1997) which found a scarcity of research demonstrating that CPD had a positive impact on patient care.

'Failure to keep up to date may lead to decay in professional knowledge and expertise and consequently to outmoded or ineffective practice' (Alsop, 1997). Continuing professional development encompasses both formal and informal learning (Eraut, 1994). This could include attending a course or undertaking a Masters programme, but also work-based learning and reflective practice. Alsop (1997) suggests that there is some evidence to show that professional education is more beneficial if it is work-based or work-related, and that it might be more effective if focused on the immediate needs of patients. This also reflects the use of problem-based scenarios in developing critical appraisal skills (Chapter 7). Continuing professional development activities need to be introduced that will facilitate decisions that can be made based on the best available evidence. In addition, involvement in clinical guidelines development, adaptation or implementation should all be recognized as part of CPD activities. The same can be said for clinical audit.

Continuing professional development: What can you do?

As managers
- Can you protect time for journal clubs, in-service sessions, library access, personal CPD such as reading and reflective practice?
- Are CPD programmes tailored for individual staff as well as for service needs?
- Do you encourage staff to record their CPD in a portfolio or equivalent?
- Do you ensure that service-wide CPD programmes have a real impact on improving care to patients?
- Do you have a system for peer review and feedback on performance?

As individuals
- How confident are you that your personal CPD programme leads to tangible improvements for patients?
- What skills enhancement do you need to include in your personal CPD programme?
- Do you record your CPD activities and their outcomes in terms of learning and practice?

Achieving quality improvement

As stated earlier, evidence-based healthcare is fundamentally about quality improvement. Identifying evidence of effectiveness is an interesting exercise, as is developing clinical guidelines and carrying out clinical audit projects. These activities can only realize their potential and recoup the time and effort invested, however, if the final step is taken in the process: that of implementing change to achieve a quality improvement. Improvements will occur by ensuring that:

- Actual practice is based on the best available evidence
- Organizational systems ensure timely and appropriate access to services for patients
- A good experience of care is provided.

A culture of commitment to excellence will ensure that ideas for improvements, or new research evidence, or new guidelines, are welcomed. Working in teams will ensure that a variety of skills are available to facilitate quality improvement (Maxwell, 1992). Individual and collective responsibility should be acknowledged and encouraged for continually finding ways to improve processes.

Achieving quality improvement: What can you do?

- Do you look for ways of improving the systems within which you work?
- What role can you play in ensuring that quality improvements result from identifying the best available evidence?
- What quality improvements have happened in your service as a result of clinical audit? How many of these have improved patients' experience of care?
- What can your colleagues contribute to achieving quality improvements?

Evidence-based healthcare: what does the future hold?

The theoretical and ethical arguments portrayed in this book, for the principle of basing decisions on the best available evidence, whether this is drawn from research, clinical expertise or patients' views and experience, are strong. Yet the evidence for improvements in services to patients that can be attributed to the high profile of evidence-based healthcare in the 1990s is limited. Is the shortage of examples of tangible benefits due to inadequacies in information systems to measure improvement, resistance to change, skills deficit, inertia, or something else? This section cannot answer these questions, but the questions already posed should help you to facilitate evidence-based healthcare. In anticipating future direction, much of the emphasis will be on implementation and change issues. The discussion will reflect on current and probable future healthcare policy, and consider how these might impact on the practicalities of service delivery for therapists.

The responsibilities of being a professional are great, in particular in protecting those who seek help, by being able to assure them of the professional's competence and the high standards of clinical practice and ethics. In the *Code of Ethics and Professional Conduct for Occupational*

Therapists (College of Occupational Therapists, 1995), there is a clear statement about the need to keep abreast of current evidence of effectiveness, in order to ensure high-quality services for patients. It states, 'occupational therapists shall be personally responsible for actively maintaining and developing their personal professional competence, and shall base service delivery on accurate and current information in the interests of high quality care'. A later section of the same document goes further, 'occupational therapists have a duty to ensure that wherever possible their professional practice is based upon established research findings'. The Chartered Society of Physiotherapy, in its *Rules of Professional Conduct* (1995) and the Royal College of Speech and Language Therapists, in its *Code of Ethics and Conduct* (1996), both stress the need to maintain competence to practise, and to only practise in those areas in which competence has been maintained.

The future of therapy research

Research activity in the therapy professions has not been established for as long as that of medicine. Recognizing the advances that had been made in a relatively short period of time, and the need to firmly bed therapists into the wider R&D agenda, led to a joint *Position Statement* (College of Occupational Therapists, Chartered Society of Physiotherapy and College of Speech and Language Therapists, 1994). In it, recommendations were made concerning priorities for the future development of research in the professions. These included the need for:

- Greater involvement in R&D committees and groups
- Management support to recognize and value the contribution of researchers
- Education and training
- A career infrastructure
- Greater understanding of research methodologies relevant to therapy research
- Involvement in dissemination and implementation initiatives.

The research capacity in the professions has increased since the Position Statement was produced, but therapists are still not as firmly bedded into R&D initiatives and systems as they should be for the benefit of patients (Bury, 1997, 1998).

Considerable funding is available for research, with an increasing emphasis on projects examining effectiveness. While this is to be welcomed and is fundamental to the requirements of evidence-based healthcare, there are many areas of therapy which have yet to be defined sufficiently for this type of research. Much practice is centred on packages of care and any number of combinations of individual interventions. This *black box* needs to be explored and components or models of care defined. However, it would appear that funding is less accessible for this type of research. Therapists, therefore, need to influence policy decisions concerning the nature of research commissioned and funded. Research priority-setting exercises are often carried out by major research funders prior to commissioning research. Therapists need to capitalize on these opportunities so that research is undertaken to fill the many gaps of uncertainty.

Consumer involvement in all aspects of R&D has yet to be fully embraced within healthcare research. The work of the Standing Advisory Group on Consumer Involvement in the NHS R&D Programme has stimulated exciting moves to facilitate this (NHSE, 1998). It will be interesting to see how long it takes for consumer involvement in R&D to become automatic, from framing research questions through to research implementation.

The NHS R&D programme continues to evolve, and new Service Delivery and Organization, and New and Emerging Technologies programmes are to be introduced to complement the existing Health Technology Assessment Programme (Bury, 1997; Mant, 1997). These will provide opportunities for therapists to influence the commissioning of research priorities. In addition, emphasis on cost-effectiveness is increasing to complement information on clinical effectiveness (Department of Health, 1997).

Opportunities exist to address many of the recommendations made in the 1994 *Position Statement*, but therapists need to be proactive to capitalize on them.

Making better use of the existing evidence in the future

You only have to consider the 1987 estimate that a staggering 20 000 articles on healthcare are published each year (Ad Hoc Working Group for Critical Appraisal of the Medical Literature, 1987) to hazard a guess at how much research has been undertaken, but has failed to inform healthcare. There is no way that individuals can be expected to keep up with the ever-increasing number of articles spread across an increasing number of journals. This is without considering the grey literature in existence. Yet, you are expected to keep up-to-date and to be safe, competent practitioners. At the same time, there is an expectation that all healthcare decisions should be based on the best available research evidence.

How is this mountain of information to be put to use? The wealth of information that already exists is gradually being synthesized, primarily in the form of systematic reviews and clinical guidelines. The work of the Cochrane Collaboration and the NHS Centre for Reviews and Dissemination has been particularly important in producing systematic reviews. These developments are to be welcomed, especially if they are written in a user-friendly format, which is easily understood, providing guidance on the implications of the research for practice. However, as Bannigan (1997) stressed, it is important that these endeavours result in high-quality information, providing assurances for the end-user. In doing so, stringent processes should have been followed to ensure the critical appraisal of the original research and the unbiased recommendations arising from this.

Therapists can help to ensure that relevant therapy literature is incorporated by becoming actively involved in initiatives, such as the Cochrane Collaboration.

Also, professionals have a responsibility to ensure that their research reaches the audience for whom it is targeted. Taylor (1997) highlights the problems that result from the inaccessibility of evidence, citing, in particular, dissertations written by students at undergraduate and postgraduate level, few of which are exposed to a wider audience. As Chapter 4 also suggested, researchers need to consider their target audiences when deciding on the most suitable format or media for the outputs of their research, and how they can actively work with others, such as the media, to reach wide audiences.

The NHS and beyond

Evidence-based healthcare is confined neither to state-funded healthcare, nor to the UK. Several times in this book, reference has been made to *The New NHS: Modern, Dependable* (Department of Health, 1997). This is the current government's framework for healthcare in England, with similar documents for Scotland, Wales and Northern Ireland (Scottish Office Department of Health, 1997; Welsh Office Department of Health, 1998; Department of Health and Social Services, 1998). This means that discussions concerning the future of healthcare in the UK have centred on the NHS. However, if the principles set out for the NHS of effective patient care, based on evidence, accountability, value for money and consistency, are widely accepted as the markers for quality, then the same should be said for any healthcare, no matter what the system or setting within which it is delivered, for example, education, social services, private or voluntary sector. The principles being taken forward for the NHS will be used to assist you to identify themes which will impact and need to be dealt with, in other settings and environments.

An environment that promotes improvement and professional development?
This chapter has already referred to the importance of CPD in achieving evidence-based healthcare. Professional bodies and the government are putting an increasingly high priority on the importance of CPD. This is based on a commitment and desire to raise the quality of practice of all members of the professions, thereby enhancing patient care. It is coupled with a new regulatory framework with which to protect the public. The draft specification of a new Bill, to replace the existing Professions Supplementary to Medicine Act (1960), states, 'a person's registration may be renewed, or a person may be readmitted to the Register, subject in either case to such conditions as to continuing professional development, further education and training or otherwise as may be prescribed' (Department of Health et al, 1997). Continuing professional development will become a mandatory requirement, a welcome emphasis, provided that for the NHS, opportunities for securing

resources, including time, can be grasped nationally and locally through education consortia.

Clinical governance emphasizes the responsibility that each individual healthcare professional has for delivering high quality services to patients, and provides a statutory responsibility of organizations, through the chief executive, for assuring quality.

Practitioners will therefore need to accept responsibility for developing and maintaining standards within their local organizations, based on national standards or clinical guidelines, developed by or in conjunction with professional bodies. Such standards and guidelines will be based on the best evidence of clinical and cost-effectiveness. National consistency and local responsiveness are the watchwords. This seems to support the model for developing national clinical guidelines and adapting them for local use, described in Chapter 8. However, the difficulties of local implementation have also been stressed, in Chapter 4, and should not be underestimated. Moving from opinion-based to evidence-based practice is not an easy step. It requires skills development, leadership, including opinion leaders, and strong change management to ensure ownership and commitment.

Valuing and involving staff, welcoming their ideas for service improvements, has the potential to create an environment for continuous improvement, in which many of the strategies for change management, discussed in this book and so fundamental to evidence-based healthcare, can flourish. With these principles applied locally in practice, coupled with an increasing knowledge base about the successful implementation of research findings, the potential for improving practice through the use of reliable new and existing research is significant. A quality organization has been described as having attributes which include the following (Department of Health, 1997):

- It ensures that evidence-based practice is in day-to-day use, with the information to support it
- Good practice, ideas and innovations *which have been evaluated* (added emphasis) are systematically disseminated within and outside the organization
- Leadership skills are developed at clinical team level
- Adverse events are detected, openly investigated, lessons learnt and promptly applied
- Lessons for clinical practice are systematically learnt from complaints made by patients.

Therapists, alongside other professionals, should develop a culture of improvement, using problems as opportunities. A positive culture in which the emphasis is on promoting **added value**, not defensively justifying services, will ensure that patients receive the services they need, and will also contribute to the future of the professions.

Programmes of care
The philosophy of identifying programmes, or systems, of care which are multiprofessional, cross organizational boundaries, are evidence-based,

cost-effective and patient-centred, will provide a vehicle for applying evidence-based healthcare. National standards frameworks will be applied locally, and therapists will need to be ready to highlight their contribution.

Measuring performance

The general public, as taxpayers, have a right to know how their local health service's performance stands up against the performance of other, similar services. Collecting such information is, however, fraught with difficulties, for example:

- How reliable will the data be?
- Will opportunities be found for creative counting, just as is alleged with Patient's Charter data?
- If information is simple enough to be easily collected and understood, will it hide the complexities that might provide meaningful explanations of best or worst performance, which would have the potential to lead to lessons for improvement?
- Will there be incentives for those who appear to perform averagely to strive for the excellence that their population will seek?

The principle, however, of collecting meaningful clinical information, is one that is central to evidence-based healthcare and clinical effectiveness. Such information will not only provide information about quality, but will also provide a further dimension of the outcome of evidence-based practice. An increased emphasis on the use of outcomes to measure health gain following interventions, and the impetus to collect more meaningful and purposeful clinical information, provides therapists with opportunities to develop evidence of effectiveness. While this will not be based on rigorous research evidence, it will provide some indication, if collected and used appropriately, nationally as well as locally, of the extent to which interventions have benefited patients.

In line with a culture of continuous improvement, therapists will want to learn from colleagues in other settings, through benchmarking, but accurate information (e.g. agreed definitions) will be essential for this to be used effectively.

Influencing

Therapists will need to influence a range of commissioners of services, including primary care groups and health authorities, who will hold budgets for healthcare for their population. It will be part of a professional's responsibility to ensure that information about the effectiveness and added value of therapy services is highlighted, not only to commissioners but also to provider groups and to consumers, who will have an increasingly important voice. Guidance (NHS Executive, 1995) about the importance of involving all professional groups in an advisory capacity in the work of health authorities has been implemented patchily. It will be important for therapy mangers to be able to discuss knowledgeably the state of the evidence base for their services, to explain the importance of patients' views and the contribution of knowledge gained from a range of research methodologies.

Similarly, therapists will need to influence the development of health improvement programmes, contributing information about the effectiveness of therapy services which can be matched with the needs of the local population for health improvement.

There has been much in this book already about the value of service users in influencing decisions about healthcare as individuals, and for populations. A commitment to including the perspectives of the local community and the experiences of patients in broader decision-making seems clear in the government's plans for the future (Department of Health, 1997). Professionals, too, must demonstrate commitment to the involvement of patients in decision-making, and to the provision of reliable information to facilitate this. The expectations of the public will continue to rise, becoming an ongoing challenge for health professionals working within finite resources. Patients will be increasingly well informed, and will need to be involved in discussions that try to balance effectiveness with patient preferences and resource limitations. In so doing, they will also be important influencers for change.

Summary

You should by now be well equipped to take forward the key themes that underpin evidence-based healthcare, no matter what your role within healthcare or the setting in which you work. The guiding principles should be applicable and relevant, even if the drivers for evidence-based healthcare vary. In the private sector, the medical insurance companies are in an influential position to determine which services will be covered. However, the debates that have centred on purchasing, such as rationing, and the fact that lack of evidence of effectiveness does not equate with ineffectiveness, are the same. Whether directly or indirectly, there will be a buyer, provider and user.

The ongoing development of evidence-based healthcare will present therapists with opportunities to further develop their knowledge base, make better use of existing knowledge, develop skills and understanding with which to apply evidence in practice, and influence those at a policy and commissioning level. In so doing, and in embracing the philosophy of working in partnership, rather than isolation, the health needs of the wider community, as well as patients, will be served. In this way, the rhetoric of evidence-based healthcare will become reality.

References

Ad Hoc Working Group for Critical Appraisal of the Medical Literature (1987). Academia and clinic: a proposal for more informative abstracts of clinical articles. *Ann Intern Med*, **106**, 598–604.

Alsop, A. (1997). Evidence based practice and continuing professional development. *B J Occup Ther*, **60**(11), 503–8.

Association of Chartered Physiotherapists Interested in Neurology (1998). *Clinical Practice Guidelines on Splinting Adults with Neurological Dysfunction*. Chartered Society of Physiotherapy.

Bannigan, K. (1997). Clinical effectiveness: systematic reviews and evidence-based practice in occupational therapy. *B J Occup Ther*, **60**(11), 479–83

Bury, T. (1997). Therapy involvement in NHS research and development. *B J Ther Rehabil*, **4**(12), 636–7.

Bury, T. (1998). Firm foundations. *Physiotherapy*, **84**(2), 59–60.

Chartered Society of Physiotherapy (1995). *Rules of Professional Conduct*. Chartered Society of Physiotherapy.

College of Occupational Therapists (1995). *Code of Ethics and Professional Conduct for Occupational Therapists*. College of Occupational Therapists.

College of Occupational Therapists, Chartered Society of Physiotherapy, and College of Speech and Language Therapists (1994). *Research and Development in Occupational Therapy, Physiotherapy and Speech and Language Therapy: A Position Statement*. Department of Health.

Department of Health (1997). *A New NHS: Modern, Dependable*. Stationery Office.

Department of Health and Social Services (1998). *Fit for the Future*: A Consultation Document on the Government's Proposals for the Future of the Health and Personal Social Services in Northern Ireland. Department of Health and Social Services.

Department of Health, Scottish Office Department of Health, Welsh Office, Department of Health and Social Services for Northern Ireland (1997). *The Health Professions Bill: Draft Specification*. Department of Health.

Eraut, M. (1994). *Developing Professional Knowledge and Competence*. Falmer Press.

Mant, D. (1997). New programmes, new opportunities. *South and West R&D Directorate Newsletter*, **12**, 1.

Maxwell, R. J. (1992). Dimensions of quality revisited: from thought to action. *Qual Health Care*, **1**, 171–7.

NHS Executive (1995). HSG(95)11. *Encouraging the Effective Involvement of Professionals in Health Authority Work*. Department of Health.

NHS Executive (1998). *Research: What's in it for Consumers?* 1st report of the Standing Advisory Group on Consumer Involvement in the NHS R&D Programme to the Central Research and Development Committee 1996/7. Department of Health.

Powell, A. (1997). *A Framework for Continuing Professional Development – A Feasibility Study – Final Report*. Chartered Society of Physiotherapy.

Royal College of Speech and Language Therapists (1996). *Communicating Quality*. Royal College of Speech and Language Therapists.

Scottish Office Department of Health (1997). *Designed to Care: Renewing the National Health Service in Scotland*. Stationery Office.

Taylor, M. C. (1997). What is evidence based practice? *B J Occup Ther*, **60**(11), 470–4.

Welsh Office Department of Health (1998). *NHSE Wales Putting Patients First*. Stationery Office.

Appendix 1
Checklists for critical appraisal

	Yes	No	Can't tell

A. ARE THE RESULTS OF THE STUDY VALID?

These can be used as screening questions, but you may need to revisit them later, especially in the case of qualitative research

	Yes	No	Can't tell
1. Did the research address a clearly focused issue? Was there a clear aim of the research? Is there ample description of informants or participants and the context? Are the outcomes clearly stated? Is the intervention clearly defined?			
	Comments:		
2. Was the method appropriate to the question? What was the study trying to do? Do you think the approach taken was the right one?			
	Comments:		

	Yes	No	Can't tell

	Yes	No	Can't tell
3. Was the sampling strategy appropriate and clearly explained? Did the investigators sample the most relevant range of individuals and settings applicable to their question? Was randomization used where appropriate?			
	Comments:		
4. Were all of the participants who entered the study properly accounted for at its conclusion? Were all patients followed up? Once randomized, were patients analysed in the groups to which they were assigned?			
	Comments:		

Detailed questions

	Yes	No	Can't tell
5. Is the literature review appropriate? Does it relate clearly to the purpose and focus of the research? Is it comprehensive and up-to-date? Does it draw on a range of sources?			
	Comments:		
6. Were ethical issues considered? Did the authors mention ethical consent? Were issues of confidentiality and anonymity dealt with?			
	Comments:		

	Yes	No	Can't tell
7. Were measures taken to reduce bias? Were patients, health care professionals and study personnel blind to treatment? Did the authors make their role in the research clear? Was the data independently assessed?			
	Comments:		
8. Where a control group was used for comparison (quantitative studies only): Were the groups similar at the start of the study? Aside from the experimental intervention, were the groups dealt with similarly?			
	Comments:		
9. Was there an adequate description of the method of data collection? Were valid and reliable outcome measures used? Were new tools piloted? How was the field work undertaken? Were observations or measures taken at appropriate times?			
	Comments:		
10. Were the methods for data analysis appropriate, clearly described and justified? Did they relate to the original research questions? Were the procedures for data analysis clearly described and theoretically justified? How were negative/discrepant results taken into account?			
	Comments:		

	Yes	No	Can't tell

B. WHAT CAN BE LEARNT FROM THE PAPER?

11. What are the key findings? Do the results address the research question? Are they likely to be clinically important? How large is the treatment effect for each of the defined outcomes in different groups? How precise are the results? What are the confidence intervals? What themes and concepts have emerged?	Comments:
12. Is there sufficient detail to assess the credibility of the findings? Is there enough detail to assess the author's interpretation? Have alternative explanations/theories for the results been explored and discounted? Are the findings reproducible and recognizable?	Comments:

C. WILL THE FINDINGS HELP YOU IN MAKING DECISIONS?

13. Can the findings be applied to your local population/individual patients/ healthcare setting? Will they help you to gain a greater insight into your setting, and if so, how? Are your patients similar to the study participants? Is the intervention transferable to your healthcare setting? Do you have the appropriate skills to deliver the intervention?	Comments:

	Yes	No	Can't tell
14. Were all the clinically important outcomes considered? Were there any other outcomes that you would expect the researcher to have used? If so, does this affect your decision?			
	Comments:		
15. Are the benefits worth the harms and costs? Were any adverse effects reported? Is there anything that would deter a patient, practitioner or manager from using the intervention? This may not be included in the paper, but what do you think?			
	Comments:		
Overall assessment:			

Checklist 2: review articles

	Yes	No	Can't tell

A. ARE THE RESULTS OF THE REVIEW VALID?

Screening questions

1. Did the review address a clearly focused issue? Was there a clear aim of the research? Is there ample description of informants or participants and the context? Are the outcomes clearly stated? Is the intervention clearly defined?			
	Comments:		

2. Did the authors look for the appropriate sort of papers? Were suitable studies selected to address the question? Were they of an appropriate methodology?			
	Comments:		

Detailed questions

3. Do you think important, relevant studies were included? What databases have been searched? What attempts were made by the authors to track down other relevant studies?			
	Comments:		

	Yes	No	Can't tell

	Yes	No	Can't tell
4. Did the review's authors do enough to assess the quality of the included studies? How were the individual studies appraised? Was more than one reviewer assessing the papers?			
	Comments:		
5. If the results of the review have been combined, was it reasonable to do so? Are the results of the trials all or mostly pointing in the same direction? Were the interventions similar enough? Were statistical tests used to examine heterogeneity (differences)?			
	Comments:		

B. WHAT ARE THE RESULTS?

6. What is the overall result of the review? Are results presented for all possible outcome measures? If a measure of effectiveness has been used what is the NNT (number needed to treat) or odds ratio?	Comments:
7. How precise are the results? What are the confidence intervals? How wide are they? Are they clinically important?	Comments:

	Yes	No	Can't tell

C. WILL THE FINDINGS HELP YOU IN MAKING DECISIONS?

8. Can the findings be applied to your local population/individual patients/healthcare setting?			
Will they help you to gain a greater insight into your setting, and if so, how? Are your patients similar to the study participants? Is the intervention transferable to your healthcare setting? Do you have the appropriate skills to deliver the intervention?	Comments:		
9. Were all the clinically important outcomes considered?			
Were there any other outcomes that you would expect the researcher to have used? If so, does this affect your decision?	Comments:		
10. Are the benefits worth the harms and costs?			
Were any adverse effects reported? Is there anything that would deter a patient, practitioner or manager from using the intervention? This may not be included in the paper, but what do you think?	Comments:		
Overall assessment:			

Appendix 2

Useful information sources

Bandolier

Pain Relief Clinic
The Churchill Hospital
Headington
Oxford OX3 7LJ
Tel: 01865 226 132
Fax: 01865 226 978
[http://www.jr2.ox.ac.uk/Bandolier]

Newsletter on evidence-based healthcare.

Centre for Evidence-Based Child Health

Department of Epidemiology and Biostatistics
Institute of Child Health
30 Guildford Street
London W1CN 1EH
Tel: 0171 242 9783 ext. 2606/2601
[http://www.ich.bpmf.ac.uk/ebm/ebm.htm]

Aims to increase the provision of effective and efficient child healthcare through an educational programme for health professionals.

Centre for Evidence-Based Medicine

University of Oxford
Nuffield Department of Clinical Medicine
Level 5
The Oxford Radcliffe NHS Trust
Headley Way
Headington
Oxford OX3 9DU
Tel: 01865 222 941
Fax: 01865 222 901
[http://www.jr2.ox.ac.uk/cebm]

Promotes evidence-based healthcare and provides support and resources to anyone who wants to make use of them. Development of learning resources.

Centre for Evidence-Based Social Services

University of Exeter
Amory Building
Rennes Drive
Exeter EX4 4RJ
Tel: 01392 263 323
Fax: 01392 263 324

Aims to improve the knowledge base of social work education and training, and facilitate implementation of research.

Chartered Society of Physiotherapy

14 Bedford Row
London WC1R 4ED
Tel: 0171 306 6666
Fax: 0171 306 6611
[http://www.csphysio.org.uk]

The professional, educational and trade union body for physiotherapists in the UK.
Advice and support on all aspects of research and clinical effectiveness in physiotherapy. National Information Resource Centre.

Clinical Effectiveness in Wales

Clinical Effectiveness Support Unit
Roseway
Llandough Hospital and Community
  NHS Trust
Penarth
Cardiff CF64 2XX
Tel: 01222 716 841
Fax: 01222 716 242

Clinical Resource and Audit Group (CRAG)

The Scottish Office
NHS Executive
St Andrew's House
Regent Road
Edinburgh EH1 3DG
Tel: 0131 2442 235
Fax: 0131 2442 683

Cochrane Collaboration

[http://hiru.mcmaster.ca/cochrane/default.htm]

See UK Cochrane Centre for further details

Preparing, maintaining and disseminating systematic reviews of the effects of healthcare.

Cochrane Collaboration
Rehabilitation and Related Therapies Field

Field Administrator
Department of Epidemiology
University of Maastricht
PO Box 616
6200 MD Maastricht
The Netherlands
Tel: +31 43 388 2394
Fax: +31 43 361 8685
[http://www-epid.unimaas.nl/html/cochrane/field.htm]

Aims to raise the profile of therapists within the Cochrane Collaboration. Coordinating searching of relevant journals.

College of Occupational Therapists

106–114 Borough High Street
London SE1 1LB
Tel: 0171 357 6480
Fax: 0171 450 2299

The professional body for occupational therapists in the UK. Information service.

Consumer Health Information Service

England and Wales
Tel: 0800 665 544
Scotland
Tel: 0800 224 488
Eastern Health and Social Services Board
Tel: 0345 581 929
Northern Health and Social Services Board
Tel: 0345 626 428
Southern Health and Social Services Board
Tel: 0800 665 544 (access local information
on this number only when dialled from
Northern Ireland)
Western Health and Social Services Board
Tel: 0800 585 329 (access only when dialled
from Northern Ireland)

Free information for healthcare professionals and users.

Critical Appraisal Skills Programme (CASP)

Institute of Health Sciences
Old Road
Headington
Oxford OX3 7LF
Tel: 01865 226 968
Fax: 01865 226 959
[http://www.ihs.ox.ac.uk/casp/]

Aims to help develop skills in the critical appraisal of evidence about effectiveness, in order to promote the delivery of evidence-based healthcare. Workshop programme.

Department of Health

Office of the Director of Research and
  Development
Richmond House
79 Whitehall
London SW1A 2NS
Fax: 0171 210 5868
[http://193.32.28.8/doh/rdd1.htm]

NHS Executive National R&D Programmes
[http://193.32.28.8/doh/rdnatprg.htm]

R&D in the Regional Offices - [http://193.32.28.8/doh/rddlinks.htm]

Information about national programmes of research and development and links to regional offices in England.

Effective Health Care Bulletins

Subscriptions Department
PO Box 77
Fourth Avenue
Harlow CM119 5BQ
Tel: 01279 623 924
Fax: 01279 639 609

Topics have included implementing clinical practice guidelines, the treatment of depression in primary care, preventing falls and subsequent injury to older people, mental health promotion in high-risk groups.

European Clearing Houses on Health Outcomes

Nuffield Institute for Health
71–75 Clarendon Road
Leeds LS2 9PL
[http://www.leeds.ac.uk/nuffield/
infoservices/ECHHO/home.html]

Aims to provide a forum for the exchange of information on the use and application of outcome measures and to increase awareness, understanding and use of outcome measurement.

Getting Research into Purchasing and Practice

Project Manager
Institute of Health Sciences
Old Road
Headington
Oxford OX3 7LF
Tel: 01865 226 724

Health Care Needs Assessments

Radcliffe Medical Press
18 Marcham Road
Abingdon
Oxon OX14 1AA
Tel: 01235 528 820
Fax: 01235 528 830

Summaries of population health care needs of a typical Health Authority (250 000) for a specific disease or population group, for example, dementia, learning difficulties, back pain and mental illness.

Health Needs Assessment

Department of Public Health and
  Epidemiology
University of Birmingham
Edgbaston
Birmingham
Tel: 0121 414 6768

Help for Health Trust

Highcroft
Romsey Road
Winchester
Hants SO22 5DH
Tel: 01962 849 100
Fax: 01962 849 079
[http://www.hfht.demon.co.uk]

Its objective is to enable people to become active partners in their own healthcare through the dissemination of high-quality information. Information service.

Kings Fund Development Centre

11–13 Cavendish Square
London W1M 0AN
Tel: 0171 307 2400
Fax: 0171 307 2801
[http://www.kingsfund.org.uk/default.htm]

The King's Fund works in a number of fields to support people's health, mainly through improving the quality of health and social care services. It includes development work in implementing clinical effectiveness and better services to carers. Provides a specialist library/ information service.

National Centre for Clinical Audit

BMA House
Tavistock Square
London WC1H 9JP
Tel: 0171 383 6451
Fax: 0171 383 6373
[http://www.ncca.org.uk]

National resource for clinical audit information. Holds a national library of audit materials and references.

National Consumer Council

20 Grosvenor Gardens
London SW1W 0DH
Tel: 0171 730 3469
Fax: 0171 730 0191

National Co-ordinating Centre for Health Technology Assessment

Boldrewood
University of Southampton
Highfield
Southampton SO16 7PX
Tel: 01703 595 586
Fax: 01703 595 639
[http://www.soton.ac.uk/~wi/hta/]

Funding for Health Technology Assessment research programme and reports of funded studies.

National Primary Care Research and Development Centre

5th Floor
Williamson Building
The University of Manchester
Oxford Road
Manchester M13 9PL
Tel: 0161 275 7601
Fax: 0161 275 7600

Funded as part of the NHS R&D Policy Research Programme.

NHS Centre for Reviews and Dissemination

University of York
Heslington
York YO1 5DD
Tel: 01904 433 634 (general enquiries)
Tel: 01904 433 707 (information service)
Fax: 01904 433 661
[http://www.york.ac.uk/inst/crd/]

For information about the DARE and NEED databases, Effective Health Care Bulletin series and systematic review reports.

NHS Public Health Development Unit

NHS Executive
Room 5E39
Quarry House
Quarry Hill
Leeds LS2 7UE
Tel: 0113 254 6128
Fax: 0113 254 6354

*Information about
nationally funded clinical
guidelines development
projects.*

Research and Development Office for the Health and Personal Social Services in Northern Ireland

12–22 Linenhall Street
Belfast BT2 8BS
Northern Ireland
Tel: 01232 553 617
Fax: 01232 553 674

Royal College of Speech and Language Therapists

7 Bath Place
Rivington Street
London EC2A 3DR
Tel: 0171 613 3855
Fax: 0171 613 3854
[http://www.rcslt.org]

*The professional body for
speech and language
therapists in the UK.*

Scottish Intercollegiate Guidelines Network

SIGN Secretariat
Royal College of Physicians of Edinburgh
9 Queen Street
Edinburgh EH2 1JQ
Tel: 0131 225 7324
Fax: 0131 225 1769
[http://pc47.cee.hw.ac.uk/sign/home.htm]

*Its objective is to improve
the effectiveness and
efficiency of clinical care
for patients in Scotland by
developing, publishing and
disseminating guidelines
that identify and promote
good clinical practice.*

The Scottish Office

Chief Scientist Office
Department of Health
NHS Executive
St Andrew's House
Regent Road
Edinburgh EH1 3DG
Tel: 0131 244 2244
Fax: 0131 244 2285

Development of research policy and funding of research policy and research programmes and projects relevant to health and the National Health Service in Scotland.

UK Clearing House on Health Outcomes

Now part of the European Clearing Houses on Health Outcomes (see above)

[http://www.leeds.ac.uk/nuffield/infoservices/UKCH/home.html]

Aimed to develop and promote approaches to health outcomes assessment within routine health care practice and to promote the role of health outcomes within decision making in health care commissioning and provision.

UK Cochrane Centre

NHS Research and Development
   Programme
Summertown Pavilion
Middle Way
Oxford OX2 7LG
Tel: 01865 516 300
Fax: 01865 516 311

Part of the Cochrane Collaboration supporting individuals in the UK. Links to review groups and fields.

[http://hiru.mcmaster.ca/cochrane/centres/UK/default.htm]

Wales Office of Research and Development for Health and Social Care

Hallinans House
22 Newport Road
Cardiff CF2 1DB
Tel: 01222 460 015
Fax: 01222 492 046

Education, training and grants for research and development.

[http://dialspace.dial.pipex.com/word/index.htm]

[http://floor.ccta.gov.uk:8080/wales/Wales.nsf]

Appendix 3

Acronyms

A&E	Accident and Emergency
ACE	Appraisal for Clinical Effectiveness
AHCPR	Agency for Health Care Policy and Research
AMED	Allied and Alternative Medicine Database
ASSIA	Applied Social Sciences Index and Abstracts
BNI	British Nursing Index
CASP	Critical Appraisal Skills Programme
CASP/few	Critical Appraisal Skills Programme Finding the Evidence Workshop
CD-ROM	Compact Disc Read Only Memory
CHiQ	Centre for Health Information Quality
CI	Confidence Interval
CINAHL	Cumulated Index to Nursing and Allied Health Literature
COT	College of Occupational Therapists
CPD	Continuing Professional Development
CSP	Chartered Society of Physiotherapy
D&C	Dilation and Curettage
DARE	Database of Abstracts of Reviews of Effectiveness
DoH	Department of Health
EBHC	Evidence-Based Healthcare
EBM	Evidence-Based Medicine
EBP	Evidence-Based Practice
EL	Executive Letter
EPOC	Cochrane Collaboration for Effective Practice and Organization of Care
GRiPP	Getting Research into Purchasing and Practice
HTA	Health Technology Assessment
ISI	Institute for Scientific Information
MeSH	Medical Subject Headings
MLA	Modern Language Association of America
NEED	NHS Economic Evaluation Database
NHS	National Health Service
NHSE	National Health Service Executive
NHSME	National Health Service Management Executive
NLM	National Library of Medicine
NNT	Number Needed to Treat
OR	Odds Ratio
PEST	Political, Economic, Sociological and Technological

R&D	Research and Development
RCSLT	Royal College of Speech and Language Therapists
RCT	Randomized Controlled Trial
ScHARR	Sheffield Centre for Health and Related Research
SD	Standard Deviation
SIGLE	System for Information on Grey Literature in Europe
SWOT	Strengths, Weaknesses, Opportunities and Threats
TENS	Transcutaneous Electrical Nerve Stimulation
UEA	University of East Anglia
WWW	World Wide Web

Index

Acronyms, 241–2
Addresses, 233–40
Allied and alternative medicine information, 115, 116, 118–19, 123, 127
AMED, 115, 116, 123, 127
Anatomy of clinical questions, 108
Applied Social Sciences Index and Abstracts, 115, 116
Appraisal, multidisciplinary, 95–6
Appraisal checklists, 151–8, 225–32
Appraisal skills, learning, 139–44
  Critical Appraisal Skills Programme, 95–6, 140–1, 237
Appraising research, 138, 149–58, 227–34
ASSIA, 115, 116
Audit, *see also* Clinical audit
  criterion-based, 195–6
  indicator-based, 196–7
  sample, 197, 199
Audit and feedback, 71–2, 81, 185

Bandolier, 121, 233
Beckhard and Harris' change model, 57–8
Behaviour change model, 77–8
Behaviour changing, 69–82
Beliefs and outcome, 14
Beliefs as evidence, 6–7
Benchmarking, 39
Best Evidence, 118
Best practice, 185–6, 192–4
BNI, 115, 116
Booklet information, 88
Books as information sources, 88–9, 112
Books on evidence-based healthcare, 122
British Library, 119
British Nursing Index, 115, 116
Business process re-engineering, 38–9

Carer Satisfaction Questionnaire, 99
Case-control studies, 145
CASP, 95–6, 140–1, 237
CD-ROM databases, 116, 117, 118, 122
Centre for Evidence-Based Child Health, 120, 235
Centre for Evidence-Based Medicine, 120, 235
Centre for Evidence-Based Social Services, 18, 235
Centre for Health Information Quality, 91
Centre for Reviews and Dissemination, 113, 240
Change:
  and the individual, 53–4
  evaluation, 62–4
  implementing, 79–80, 203–4
  interventions to facilitate, 69–76, 212
  management, 45–64
    tools and techniques, 58–61

maintaining, 81
models, 56–8, 77–8
triggers, 48–9, 77
types of, 48, 49
Changing behaviour, 69–82
Chartered Society of Physiotherapy, 118–19, 236
Checklists for appraisal, 151–8, 227–34
Child health information, 120, 235
CINAHL, 115, 116, 123, 127
Citizens' juries, 95
Clearing Houses on Health Outcomes, 238, 242
Clinical audit, 166, 182–205
  achieving change, 202–4
  acting on the findings, 202–4
  confidentiality, 202
  criterion-based, 195–6
  data collection, 200–1
  definitions of, 183–4
  evidence-based, 186–8
  findings, 201–2
  guideline implementation, 166, 186
  indicator-based, 196–7
  National Centre, for 113, 240
  objectives, 192
  presenting findings, 201–2
  re-audits, 185, 204
  results, 201, 202
  sample size, 197, 199
  specialized staff for, 188
  stages of, 184, 187–8, 189–204
  team *vs* individual, 189
  topic choice, 189–92
Clinical benefit, 148–9
Clinical decision support systems, 75
Clinical effectiveness, 26–41, 186
  stakeholders, 30–6
Clinical Effectiveness in Wales, 236
Clinical expertise and decision making, 10–11, 17
Clinical expertise as evidence, 6
Clinical governance, 220
Clinical guidelines, 162–80, 185–6
  changing behaviour, 70, 164, 178, 194–5
  compliance, 195–201
  definitions of, 162, 185–6
  desirable attributes of, 173–4
  developing, 96, 164, 169–74, 214
  disseminating, 175
  economic factors, 165, 170
  implementing, 70, 166, 175–9, 194–5
  importance of, 163–5
  legal aspects, 167–9
  local implementation, 177–9

Clinical guidelines (*cont.*)
   local *vs* national, 174–9
   presentation format, 173
   professional bodies, 179–80
   use by patients, 165
   use by purchasers, commissioners, 167
   uses of, 163–7
Clinical questions, anatomy of, 108
Clinical Resource and Audit Group, 236
Clinical significance, 148
Cochrane Centres, 112, 113, 242
Cochrane Collaboration, 112, 236–7
Cochrane Controlled Trials Register, 117–18
Cochrane Database of Systematic Reviews, 117
Cochrane Library, 117–18, 127–30
Cohort studies, 145–6
Collaboration, 213
College of Occupational Therapists, 119, 237
Commissioner-professional relationship, 33–4
Commissioning, evidence–based, 5, 19–20, 21–2, 33
Commissioning decisions, 19–20, 33
   use of clinical guidelines, 167
Complaints, use of, 191–2
Computer software:
   clinical decision support systems, 75
   reference management, 131–3
Conference proceedings, finding, 122
Conferences, 73
Confidence intervals, 148
Confirmation of change, 81
Consensus development, 75, 172
Consumer Council, National, 240
Consumer Health Information Services, 89, 237
Consumers, 31–3, *see also* Patients
Continuing professional development, 35, 130–1, 136–7, 166,
   217–18, 222–23
Controlled clinical trials, 145
Cost-benefit analysis, 36–7, 165
Cost-effectiveness, 30–1
Criterion-based audit, 195–6
Critical appraisal:
   checklist, 151–8, 227–34
   learning, 139–44
   multidisciplinary, 95–6
   of research, 138, 149–58, 227–34
   Skills Programme, 95–6, 140–1, 237
Cumulated Index to Nursing and Allied Health Literature,
   115, 116, 123, 127
Current awareness publications, 123

DARE, 113, 118
Database of Abstracts of Reviews of Effectiveness, 113, 118
Databases, 113–18, 122
   access to, 116
   allied and alternative medicine, 115, 116, 119, 123, 127
   AMED, 115, 116, 123, 127
   ASSIA, 115, 116
   Best Evidence, 118
   BNI, 115, 116

CD-ROM, 116, 117, 118, 122
   choosing, 110–11, 113–14
   CINAHL, 115, 116, 123, 127
   Cochrane Library, 117–18, 123, 127–30
   comparing, 123–30
   DARE, 113, 118
   EMBASE, 115, 116, 123, 124–6
   filters, 116–17
   general, 114–17
   grey literature, 122
   Internet, 113, 116, 122, 127–30
   MEDLINE, 114, 116, 117, 123, 124–6
   NEED, 113
   online, 116
   printed, 116
   search strategies, 111, 113–18, 123–30
   SIGLE, 122
   social sciences, 115, 116
   specialist, 114, 117–18
   worked examples using, 123–30
Decision making, evidence-based, 10–11, 14, 19, 20
Decision making by patients, 9–11, 14, 31–2, 86–8, 165
Decision making by professionals, 10–11, 14, 16–17, 86–8
Department of Health:
   clinical effectiveness initiative, 28–30
   Research and Development Strategy, 3–4, 17–18, 28
Diffusion of research, 67–8
DISCERN, 91
Dissemination of research, 68, 69
   NHS Centre for reviews and, 113, 240

Economics and clinical effectiveness, 30–1, 36–7
Economics of guideline development, 165, 170
Education:
   acquiring appraisal skills, 139–44
   changing behaviour, 70–6
   continuing professional development, 35, 130–1, 136–7,
   217–18, 222–23
Effective Health Care Bulletins, 238
Effectiveness, clinical, 26–41, 186
Efficacy, 26
EMBASE, 115, 116, 123, 124–6
EndNote Plus, 132
Ethics:
   change management, 61–2
   equity of care, 37–8
   purchasing policy, 33
   wasting resources, 37
Ethnography, 146
European Clearing Houses on Health Outcomes, 238
Evidence-based commissioning, 5, 19–20, 21–2, 33
Evidence-based decision making, 10–11, 14, 19, 20
Evidence-based healthcare:
   advantages of, 23
   barriers to, 22–3
   books on, 122
   centres for, 120, 235
   describing, 4–5
   journals on, 121

opportunities offered, 22–3
Evidence-based management, 5, 21
Evidence-based medicine, 6, *see also* Evidence-based
    healthcare
Evidence Based Medicine, 121
Evidence-based patient choice, 5, 10–11
Evidence-based patient information, 90–3
Evidence-based policy, 5, 17–18
Evidence-based practice, 5, 6–16
    evaluating, 166
    implementing, 166
Evidence-based purchasing, 5, 19–20, 21–2, 33–4, 167
Evidence sources, 6–11, 109–23, 163–5
Executive Letters on clinical effectiveness, 29
Experimental design, *see* Research methods
Exposure, 108

Filters, 116–17
Finding the evidence, 107–35
    clinical guidelines, 171–2
    worked examples, 123–30
Focus groups, 91, 94–5
Force field analysis, 59–60

Getting Research into Purchasing and Practice, 238
Government initiatives, 28–9
Grey literature, 122
GRiPP, 238
Grounded theory, 146
Guidelines, 162–80
    changing behaviour, 70, 164, 178, 194–5
    compliance, 195–201
    definitions of, 162, 185–6
    desirable attributes of, 173–4
    developing, 96, 164, 169–74, 214
    disseminating, 175
    economic factors, 165, 170
    implementing, 70, 166, 175–9, 194–5
    importance of, 163–5
    legal aspects, 167–9
    local *vs* national, 174–9
    presentation format, 173
    professional bodies, 179–80
    use by patients, 165
    use by purchasers, commissioners, 167
    uses of, 163–7

Hawthorne effect, 153
Health, Department of:
    clinical effectiveness initiative, 28–30
    Research and Development Strategy, 3–4, 17–18, 28
Health Care Needs Assessments, 238
Health Information Services, 89, 237
Health Needs Assessment, 239
Healthcare, inequalities in, 37–8
Help for Health Trust, 239

Implementing guidelines, 70, 166, 175–9, 194–5
Implementing research, 68–9, 79–80

Indicator-based audit, 196–7
Individual *vs* population needs, 21–2
Inequalities in healthcare, 37–8
Influencing others, 221
Information for patients, 31–2, 86–93
Information sources:
    addresses of, 235–42
    books, 88–9, 112, 122
    current awareness publications, 123
    databases, 113–18, 122
    grey literature, 122
    Internet, 89, 113, 116, 120, 121, 122
    journals, 112, 120–1
    leaflets, 32, 88–9
    libraries, 109–10, 111–12, 119
    specialist centres, 112–13, 118–19
    support groups, 89
    verbal information, 90
    videos, 92
Integrated care pathways, 40–1
Interactive video, 92
Internet, evidence-based information on, 89, 120, 121
Internet, databases on the, 113, 116, 122
    worked example using, 123, 127–30
Internet use by patients, 89
Internet Web sites, 113, 116, 120, 121, 234–42
    worked example using, 123, 127–30
Intervention, 108

Journal articles:
    appraising, 138, 149–58, 227–34
    as evidence sources, 112, 120–1
    filing, 131–3
    importance of, 137
    interpreting results of, 147–9, 150
    structure of, 149–51
Journal clubs, 142–4
Journals on evidence–based healthcare, 121

King's Fund, 237

Leaflet, patient information, 32, 88–9
Lewin's change model, 56–7
Libraries, 109–10, 111–12, 119
    Cochrane, 117–18, 127–30
    guides to, 110
Library Master, 133
Literature searches, 111, 113–18, 123–30
Longitudinal studies, 145–6

Management, evidence-based, 5, 21
Managing change, 45–64
Marketing and changing behaviour, 75–6
Media campaigns, 74
MEDLINE, 114, 116, 117, 123, 124–6
Meta-analysis, 146, 149
Multidisciplinary teams:
    change management, 51–3
    critical appraisal by, 95–6

Multidisciplinary teams (*cont.*)
   difficulties with, 96–7
   evidence-based practice, 15
   importance of, 15, 213–14
   integrated care pathways, 40–1

National Centre for Clinical Audit, 113, 240
National Consumer Council, 240
National Co-ordinating Centre for Health Technology
   Assessment, 240
National Health Service:
   Centre for Reviews and Dissemination, 113, 240
   clinical effectiveness initiative, 28–30
   Economic Evaluations Database, 113
   Public Health Development Unit, 241
   Research and Development Strategy, 3–4, 17–18, 28
National Primary Care Research and Development Centre,
   240
NEED, 113
NHS Centre for Reviews and Dissemination, 113, 240
NHS Economic Evaluations Database, 113
NHS Public Health Development Unit, 241
Northern Ireland, Research and Development Office, 241
Numbers needed to treat, 149
Nursing databases, 115, 116

Occupational Therapists, College of, 119, 237
Odds ratio, 149
Online databases, 116
Opinion leaders, 73–4, 80
Opinions and consensus development, 75
Opinions as evidence, 9
Outcome and beliefs, 14
Outcome information, 238, 242
Outcome measures, 99
Outreach visits, 72–3

P values, 148
PAPYRUS, 132
Patient complaints, 191–2
Patient focus groups, 91, 94–5
Patient-mediated interventions, 74
Patient-professional relationship, 10–11, 14, 32, 86–8, 90, 93
Patient responsibilites, 32–3
Patient surveys, 94
Patients:
   decision making by, 9–11, 14, 31–2, 86–8, 165
   evidence-based choice, 5
   evidence from, 6–7
   guideline development, 96, 164, 170, 171, 214
   information for, 31–2, 86–93
   involvement, 213
   obtaining views of, 94–6, 191
   policy decisions, 93–7
   questions asked by, 86
   research involvement, 98–100
   support groups, 89
Patient's Charter, 31
People categories, 78

Performance measures, 39, 221
PEST analysis, 61
Phenomenology, 146
Physiotherapy, Chartered Society of, 118–19, 236
Policy, evidence-based, 5, 17–18
Policy decisions, patient involvement, 93–7
Politicians promoting evidence-based healthcare, 30–1
Population *vs* individual needs, 21–2
Position Statement, professionals body, 219–20
Practice, evidence-based, 5, 6–16
Primary care, 18, 71
Problem-based learning, 139–40
ProCite, 133
Professional bodies:
   addresses, 236, 237, 241
   guideline development, 179–80
   Position Statement, 219–20
   role of, 35–6, 139–40
   rules of conduct, 217
Professional development, 35, 130–1, 136–7, 215–16, 219–20
Professional-patient relationship, 10–11, 14, 32, 86–8, 90, 93
Professional-purchaser relationship, 33–4
Professional responsibilities, 35, 216–7
Professional rules of conduct, 219
Professionals, treatment choice by, 10–11, 107–8
Professionals' behaviour, changing, 69–82, 93, 178
Prompt systems, 75
Protocols, 185–6 *see also* Guidelines
Public opinions, 94, 95
Purchaser-professional relationship, 33–4
Purchasing, evidence-based, 5, 19–20, 21–2, 33
Purchasing decisions, 19–20, 33
   use of clinical guidelines, 167

Qualitative *vs* quantitative research, 144–5
Quality, 27–8, 184, 218–19
Quality impact analysis, 189–91
Questionnaires, 94, 99

Randomized controlled trials, 9, 145
Rationing healthcare, 20
Readiness for change, 77–8
Reading time, organizing, 130–1, 136–7
Re-engineering, 38–9
Reference Manager, 132
References, filing, 131–3
Reminder systems, 75
Reports, finding information about, 122
Research aims, 7
Research appraisal, 138, 149–58, 227–34
Research articles:
   appraising, 138, 149–58, 227–34
   filing, 131–3
   importance of, 137
   interpreting results of, 147–9, 150
   structure of, 149–51
Research as evidence, 6, 7–9, 112, 120–1
Research diffusion and dissemination, 67–8, 69
Research implementation, 68–9, 79–80

Research involving patients, 98–100, 218
Research methods, 7–9, 144–6
    case-control, 145
    cohort studies, 145–6
    controlled clinical trials, 145
    ethnography, 146
    grounded theory, 146
    longitudinal studies, 145–6
    meta-analysis, 146, 149
    phenomenology, 146
    qualitative *vs* quantitative, 144–5
    randomized controlled trials, 9, 145
    reviews, 8–9
    systematic reviews, 8–9, 146
Research results, interpreting, 147–9, 150
Responsibility charting, 60–1
Reviews, 8–9
    systematic, 8–9, 146
Royal College of Speech and Language Therapists, 241

Scottish Intercollegiate Guidelines Network, 241
Scottish Office, 241
Search strategies, 111, 113–18, 123–130
Service users, *see* Patients
SIGLE, 122
Social marketing, 75–6
Social sciences database, 115, 116
Social services, 18
    Centre for Evidence-Based, 18, 235
Software:
    clinical decision support systems, 75
    reference management, 131–3
Speech and Language Therapists, Royal College of, 241
Stakeholder analysis, 60
Stakeholder conferences, 94
Stakeholders, 30–6
Standards, 185–6, *see also* Guidelines
Statistics, 147–9
    clinical significance, 148

confidence intervals, 148
    descriptive, 147
    inferential, 148
    meta-analysis, 149
    numbers needed to treat, 149
    odds ratio, 149
    purpose, 147
Stroke care, 37–8
Support groups, 89
Surveys, 94, 99
SWOT analysis, 61
System for Information on Grey Literature in Europe, 122
Systematic reviews, 8–9, 146

Telephone help lines, 89
Textbooks as information sources, 112
Textbooks on evidence–based healthcare, 122
Theses, finding information about, 122
Treatment choice, 10–11, 107–8
Treatment variations, 37–8

UK Clearing House on Health Outcomes, 242
UK Cochrane Centre, 112, 242
Uncertainty, dealing with, 16–17
Users, *see* Patients
Users' Guides, 121

Variations, reducing, 165–6
Verbal information, 90
Video information, 92

Wales:
    Clinical Effectiveness Support Unit, 236
    Research and Development Office, 242
Web sites, 113, 116, 120, 121, 234–42
    worked example using, 123, 127–30
Working groups, 46–7
Workshops, 73, 95–6, 141–2